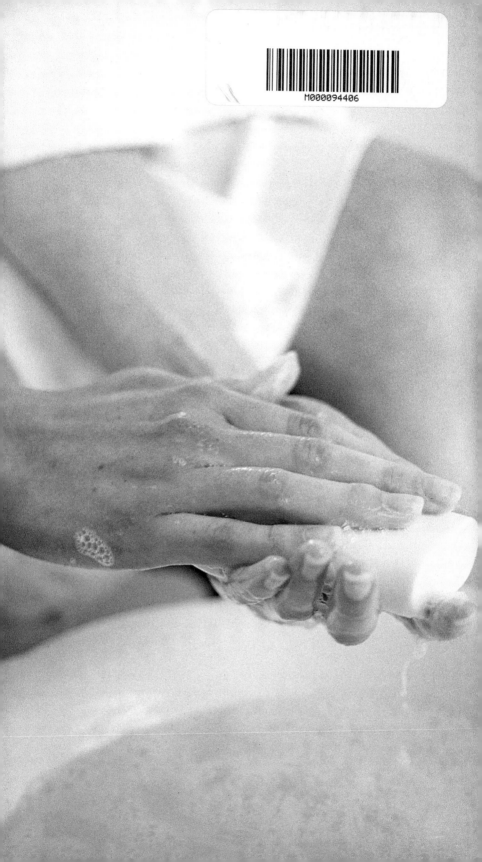

aromatiQues

a sensualist's guide to aromatic oils

Éva-Marie Lind

Photography by Robert Olding

SOMA
san francisco

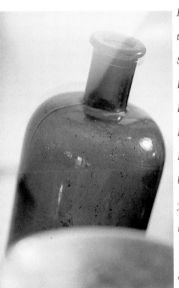

In the words of my author friend Lee Williams, no task is truly accomplished alone. A select and special thank you to Seza Magdalena Eccles, Krishna Madappa, Kent McKay, Drew Lightfoot, Lynn Ann Kister, Jennifer Edwards, Felicity Lawrence, Gabriel Mojay, Rachael Shapiro, Ixchel Leigh, Dr. Michael Sears, Jadyne Reichner, Charley and Ginny Hoppe, and Robert Clay Shiveley, for entering my world and becoming a part of my extended family. I thank you for your continued friendship, support, guidance, love, and inspiration to my work and my life.

Thank you to my editors Beth Weber, Laura leGrand, and Floyd Yearout, who supported my neuroses and my enthusiasms, and with unrelenting cheer and against all odds saw this small book to its celebrated completion. Thank you also to Cliff Morgan, Robert Olding, Erika Sloan, Amy Armstrong, and James Connolly.

A special thank you to Aromatherapy Quarterly *and* The American Alliance of Aromatherapy News Quarterly, *which were the first to publish my aromatic writings and recipes.*

This book is lovingly dedicated

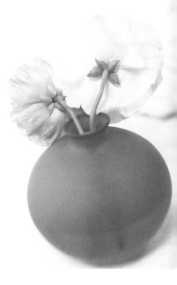

to Courtney Brianne.

PLEASE NOTE:

Aromatiques is not sponsored by or affiliated with any other entity using Aromatique in its product or company name, and this publisher is not engaged in the manufacture or sale and does not endorse or recommend specific aromatic products.

This book was created as an introduction to the world of aromatherapy. The ingredients, recipes, and uses we present should be viewed as a supplement to, not a substitute for, professional treatment or medical care. The essential oils discussed here should not be used in the treatment of a medical condition or in a therapy without consulting a qualified healthcare professional. The author and publisher cannot be held responsible for mishap resulting from the misuse of either essential oils or of any methods mentioned in this book.

SOMA Books is an imprint of Bay/SOMA Publishing, Inc. 555 De Haro St., No. 220, San Francisco, CA 94107.

Copy Editor: Stacey Lynn
Proofreader: Virginia
  Simpson-Magruder
Designer: Level

Library of Congress Cataloging-in-Publication data
Lind, Éva-Marie.
  Aromatiques: a sensualist's guide to aromatic oils/ Éva Marie Lind: photography by Robert Olding.
    p. cm.
  ISBN 1-57959-069-1
  1. Aromatherapy, I. Title
RM666,A68L56 1999
615' .321—dc21
99-3759 CIP

Printed in China
10 9 8 7 6 5 4 3 2 1

Distributed by Publishers Group West

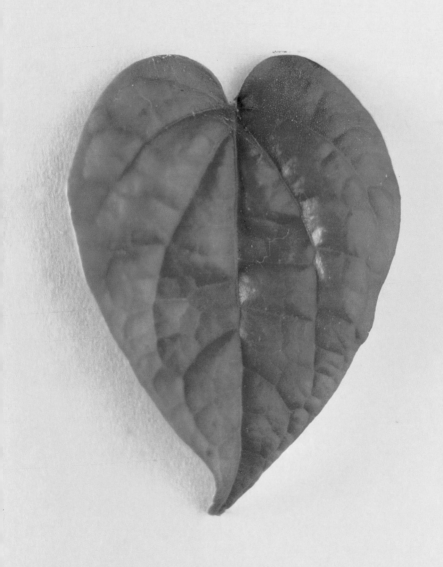

contents

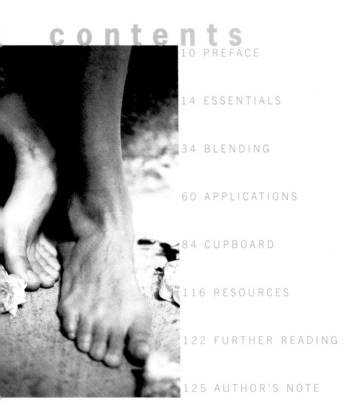

"Show me your garden, provided it be your own,
—Alfred Austin

Preface

The day was marked by a fine summer's rain, and now, as dusk
descends, a warm mist rises from the mossy stones of my garden
pathway, like the evening lifting her skirts. I meander barefoot
out onto the damp, clover-laced grass, as the pungent earth wafts
unparalleled melodies of scent upward to encircle me. Night-blooming
tuberose, star lilies, and jasmine lift their pale white faces, and I lift
my own, to the diffuse pale blue light of the moon.

In the encroaching coolness the flowers are just beginning to
add a sweet fragrant fringe to the breeze, a scent that holds for me
hints of ripe peaches and plums, ready to fall to the ground if the
wind were to tickle them sufficiently. My nose picks up a variety of
scented geranium, chamomile, rosemary, thyme, lavender, and sage,
all giving up their exhausted scents with the moistening of the earth.
I am keenly aware of a feathered moth on her nightly journey, who has
left her scent through the brushing of pollen dust upon my surprised
cheek. Amazing to think that such a fragile creature has the ability to
smell its own mate miles away!

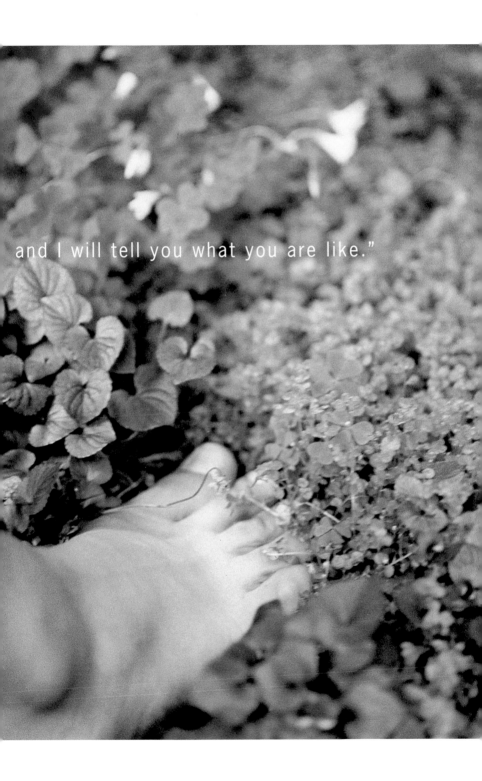

and I will tell you what you are like."

I fear that words are inadequate to describe what I have been blessed to experience in this moment. As I mature in years, I seek to stretch my vocabulary, for to me words are companions rather than mere segments of characters and syllables. And every time I am introduced to a wonderful new aroma, I make a point to revel in my sense of smell, just as I did as a small child. The sentiments of Walter Hubert come to my mind. In *Naked Flowers Exposed* (HarperCollins, 1997) he professed, "Now that I am older and almost ready to face the world, I look back on my youth and wonder if I will ever be able to smell the world in the same way again."

Webster's dictionary profoundly yet simply defines "breathe" as "to live." I cannot bear to imagine life without scent. Our sense of smell acts as a portal to the deepest levels of our subconscious mind. It is deftly linked to our individual personalities and histories. Even a simple walk down a garden path may unleash a host of associations and memories.

Although botanical essences are blessed with distinctive aromatic characteristics, it is important to keep in mind that they are not only fragrant. Just as they afford protection and healing for the botanical hosts from which they are extracted, their chemical makeup supports our vital organs while their scent balances our minds and emotions, helping us to sustain optimal health and quality of life.

There once was an age when the division between food, medicine, and botanicals did not exist. People relied on what they found in the fields and forests and on the bounty of their herb and flower beds for relief from hunger, malaise, and injury. Aromatic botanicals were not enjoyed for their scent alone; they had a physical and psychological purpose as well. Technology has thrown us into an era in which we depend more on what is conceived, concocted, and made readily and conveniently available to us than on what the earth provides for us. Essential oils and aromatherapy have been part of our cultural heritage for thousands of years, and although their mysteries have lain dormant in many respects, we are once again beginning to realize their potential.

For the art and science of aromatherapy to be adequately represented, several vast and descriptive volumes would be necessary. This book is presented to you, its reader, merely as an introduction and a celebratory portrait, a fragment compiled from a far greater landscape. But as you browse these pages, it is my hope that your curiosity will be piqued to explore what I feel could be one of the most influential, enhancing, and profound experiences of your life.

May the essences not only alleviate your physical ailments, may they heighten the wisdom and focus of your mind, bring joy and sunshine to your soul, put renewed lightness and energy into your step, and reawaken sensuality in your heart.

ÉVA-MARIE LIND

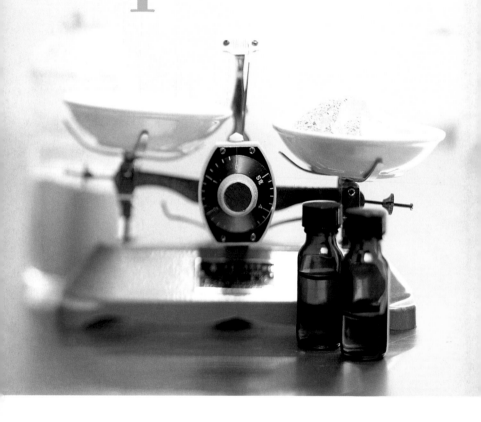

e₁ssentials

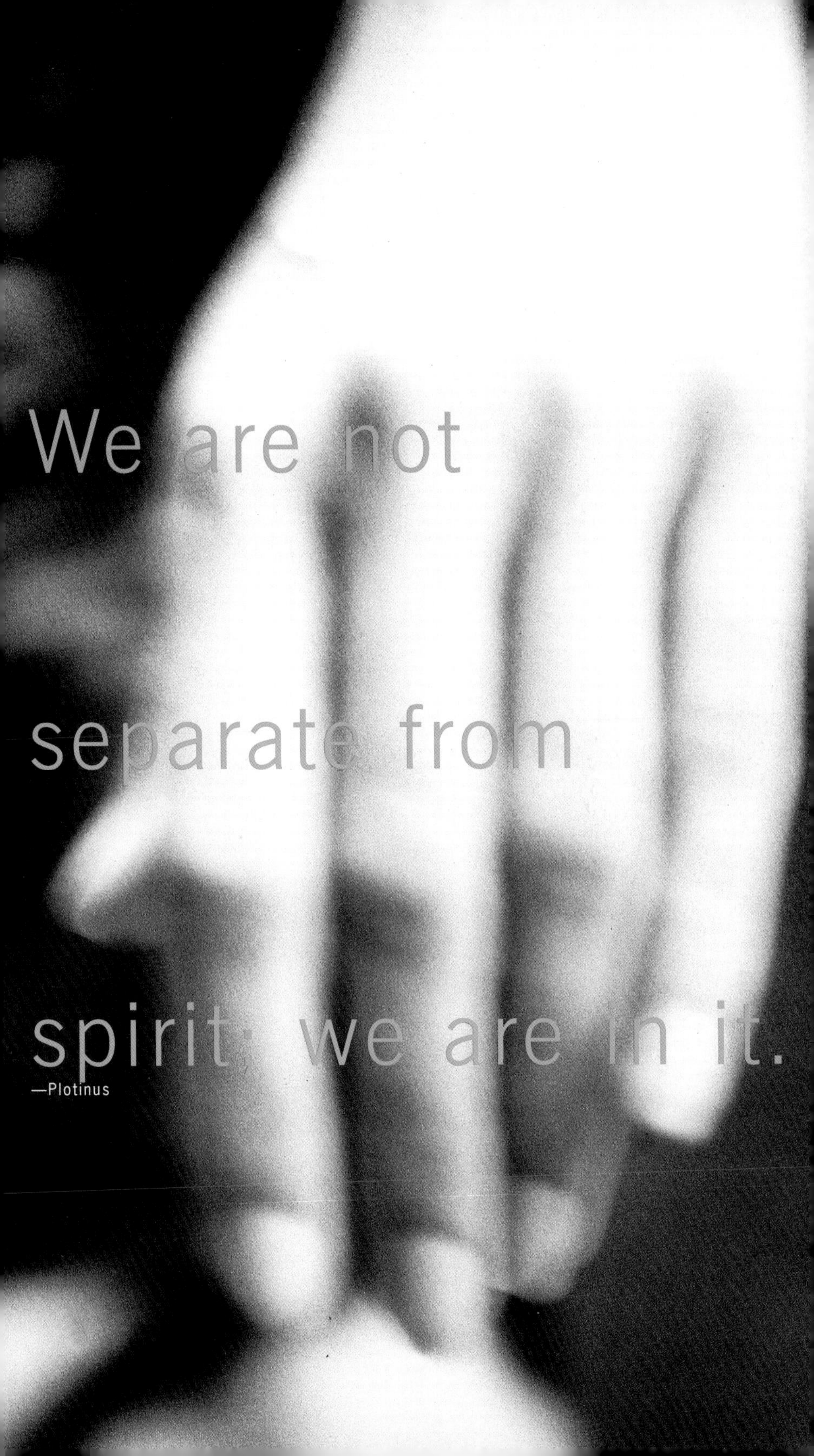

We are not

separate from

spirit: we are in it.
—Plotinus

An essential oil could be simply defined as the

concentration of a multitude of volatile molecules that are responsible

for the fragrance and health of the aromatic botanical host in which

they were created. The word *volatile* is derived from the Latin *volare*,

"to fly," and volatile molecules evaporate quite readily at normal

atmospheric pressures and at room temperature. This is what makes

their fragrance so wonderfully perceptible to us.

Every blade of grass has its angel that

An aromatic essential oil resides in specialized secretory glands within its botanical host. These glands can be housed in roots, rhizomes, stems and stalks, heartwood, bark and wood, gums and resins, rind (peel), seeds, fruits, nuts or berries, twigs, leaves, and, ultimately and supremely, in flowers. Essential oils (also called "essences") construct for their botanical hosts an unparalleled immune system through their naturally occurring antibiotics, hormones, vitamins, and antiseptic qualities. An aromatic plant ultimately relies on its fragrant components for support and health.

bends over it and whispers, grow, grow.
—the Talmud

We, likewise, rely on botanicals, whether medicinal, culinary, or aromatic, to enhance our quality of life and maintain our sense of well-being. You may be surprised to learn that out of 600,000 plant species, only about 5 percent have been thoroughly investigated and recognized for their aromatic and medicinal advantages. Theoretically, what an essential oil is able to extend to us in health support can be compared to what it affords its botanical host. The oil's therapeutic properties depend on its individual molecular components and can include analgesic, antiseptic, antiviral, anti-inflammatory, anti-spasmodic, aphrodisiac, bactericidal, viricidal, fungicidal, digestive, diuretic, nervine, hyper/hypotensive, regenerative, sedative, stimulant, and tonic properties—and that's just the start of the list!

The quality and strength of an essential oil varies in relation to the plant species, the richness of the soil in which the plant was grown, the climate, the method of cultivation, the time and method of harvest, and the process of distillation. Lavender grown at a high altitude, for example, produces an essential oil with a high ester standard, in particular the ester of linalyl acetate, for which lavender is often sought. The composition of an essential oil depends on the part of the plant that has been harvested and distilled. For instance, bitter orange produces three different aromatic oils: neroli from its blossoms, petitgrain from its leaves, and bitter orange from its peel. The season, the weather conditions, and even the time of day are all important factors in deciding when to extract an essential oil.

At least 75 percent of all essential oils are obtained by a distillation method. In general, this is a lengthy process that can take 48 hours or more and can be energy intensive, involving wood, gas, and electricity. Distillation works to isolate the water-insoluble, volatile components of the plant. Heat from the process can change the natural composition of the oil and may even manufacture new and beneficial components. For example, the distillation of chamomile produces *chamazulene*, a valuable anti-inflammatory component.

Some of the more fragile flower components and fragrances are damaged by heat and can be captured only through solvent extraction. This method produces semisolid materials called "concretes," which are valued by perfumers. When concretes undergo a further refining process, they become "absolutes." Usually rich in color and of a more viscous consistency than distilled essential oils, absolutes often retain some of the chemicals used to extract them. For this reason, many aromatherapists choose not to incorporate them into their therapies. The natural resin of trees is often extracted with solvents (though frankincense and some other resins can also be produced by distillation). These products are called "oleoresins," "resinoids," and "balsams."

A few essential oil extracts are still produced laboriously by hand, using ancient traditional methods such as enfleurage, maceration, and cold expression. These oils, which can include tuberose, jasmine, and certain citrus oils produced in the Mediterranean, are precious and often very expensive. The method of extraction and the care taken in the process are vitally important to the pristine quality as well as the "personality" and chemical structure of an aromatic essential oil.

It is important for the buyer to be aware that even after the plant material undergoes distillation, the essential oil may be further altered, refined, "rectified," "folded," or "fractionated" to obtain several grades of oil. In the flavoring and perfume industries, this is done to remove impurities or components that are reputed to be irritating or harmful. In aromatherapy practice, these alterations are thought to disrupt the harmony of the essential oil; these oils are generally not accepted by the therapist.

The chemical composition of an essential oil is quite complex. Essential oils are abundant in oxygenated compounds such as aldehydes, alcohols, esters, ketones, oxides, and phenols and hydrocarbons, which include terpenes, monoterpenes, sesquiterpenes, and minute quantities of hemiterpenes and diterpenes. The chemical components of oils relate directly to their therapeutic actions. If you know that an essential oil is high in terpenes, for example, as many citrus oils are, then you know that it will function well as an anti-inflammatory or bactericide. If it has a sufficient range of alcohols, such as with lavender, geranium, or rose, it will generally be both nontoxic and antiviral.

Furthermore, the percentage of such components can dictate the health and shelf life of an essential oil. Since terpenes are unsaturated hydrocarbons and absorb oxygen from the air, oils high in terpenes (such as citrus and conifers) are susceptible to spoilage. Esters undergo partial hydrolysis and can turn acidic, so oils high in esters (such as lavender) can spoil if stored improperly. The quality of oils high in aldehydes (such as lemongrass) can diminish over time, while oils high in terpene alcohols (such as geranium) are relatively stable for long periods. Some oils (such as peppermint) can also "resinificate," becoming more viscous with time, while others (such as vetiver and ylang ylang) mature like fine wines.

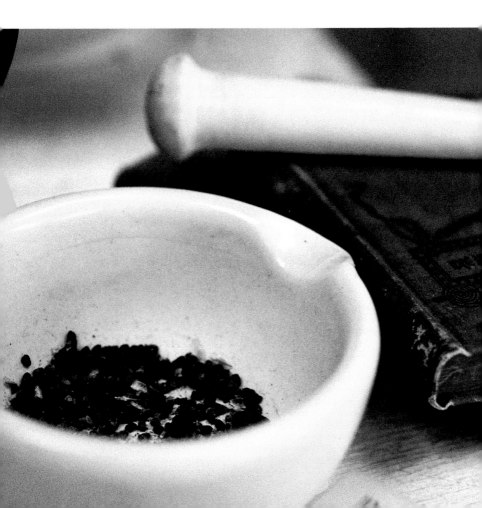

"Nature identical" is a term used primarily in the pharmaceutical and perfumery industries and refers to oils that are not obtained by natural distillation methods but rather are replicated synthetically. Such oils by no means contain the vital energy and naturally occurring therapeutic chemical composition of true essential oils. They serve no purpose for therapy but instead afford a means for the "regularity" in scent required by the cosmetic, food, pharmaceutical, and perfumery industries.

It has become highly fashionable to obtain essential oils with the "organic" label attached to them. However, stringent guidelines for producing organic essential oils have yet to be firmly established in much of the world. Furthermore, most aromatic botanicals are grown, harvested, and produced in countries that rarely have the resources to incorporate pesticides and herbicides into their manufacturing of botanicals, and therefore "organic" production is not necessarily an indicator of purity.

"Ethically wildcrafted" botanicals are labeled such because they are formulated from indigenous plants that grow wild, without the use of fertilizers, insecticides, and other chemicals. This is the case with many lavenders, which are believed to produce their own insecticides.

"Ecologically sensible" is how many companies describe their cultivated organic oils, whether they are rigidly certified or not. Many of the better suppliers include their organic oils in this category.

Some essential oils actually season and mature with age. Many of these oils, such as frankincense and sandalwood, are obtained from plants that take a good deal of time to aromatically mature. A number of companies now deal in these aged, "vintage" oils.

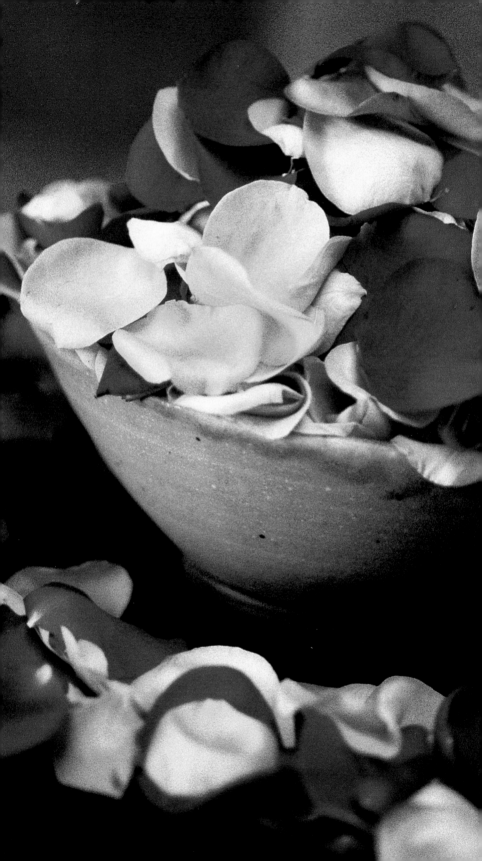

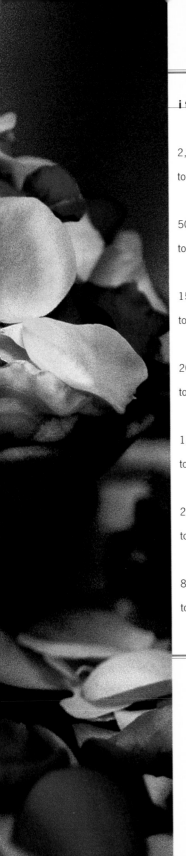

2,000 rose petals
to make 1 drop of essential oil

50 to 100 pounds of eucalyptus leaves
to make 1 pound of essential oil

150 to 250 pounds of lavender tops
to make 1 pound of essential oil

200 to 300 pounds of rosemary
to make 1 pound of essential oil

1,000 to 1,500 pounds of chamomile heads
to make 1 pound of essential oil

2,500 to 4,500 pounds of jasmine blooms
to make 1 pound of absolute

8,000 to 10,000 pounds of melissa flowers
to make 1 pound of essential oil

BUYING ESSENTIAL OILS

To determine whether the oil you are purchasing is of the highest quality and purity, it helps to know as much as possible about it. Along with understanding the origin and extraction method of the oil you are purchasing, being aware of the reputation of the company you are dealing with is of utmost importance. Insist that your supplier work with manufacturers who will ensure that their essential oils are of aromatherapeutic quality: 100 percent pure, unaltered, undiluted, nonsynthetic botanical distillates and extracts. Essential oils used in their "whole" form are less likely to cause irritation than oils with their constituents removed.

We live in a day of "buyer beware," but rather than look upon this as a burden, add it to the adventure of exploration and personal empowerment. Here are some tips for judging the quality of an essential oil.

quality tips

- Be sure to buy only essential oils that are labeled "pure aromatherapy grade."

- Purchase essential oils only in undyed, integrated-color (usually amber, cobalt blue, or violet) glass bottles without droppers.

- To smell the oil, place a drop on a tissue rather than smelling directly from an open bottle. Its aroma after it has been exposed to the air is more indicative of its true scent.

- Drop the oil onto a professional perfume blotter strip or white, unbleached, semiporous paper. A drop of essential oil on paper should leave a waterlike stain, not an oil ring. A few oils (such as blue chamomile or red mandarin) will stain white paper.

- An essential oil should leave no oily residue on the skin. It should absorb quickly and leave the skin feeling silky. If possible, before purchasing an essential oil, do a skin patch test (see page 31).

- An essential oil touched to the tip of your tongue should not have an alcohol or chemical taste to it.

- If you know your essential oil well by its Latin nomenclature, you will know what you are paying for. A lavender is not just a lavender, a marjoram not just a marjoram. Oils obtained from different species have different qualities.

- Be aware of misleading terminology: The words "oil of," particularly when pertaining to more costly botanicals such as rose, sandalwood, or jasmine, could mean a maceration of plant material in vegetal oil or even a synthetic perfume oil. This term is a definite warning sign.

- The adulteration most difficult to uncover is the oil with added natural or synthetic dilutants and stretchers, such as the odorless and tasteless DEP and DPG. These additions may be blended into the oil or even added to the plant material before distillation. The results of chemical analyses of the oil, usually available at the buyer's request, will reveal these additions but can be quite difficult for the layperson to interpret. More helpful to the novice purchaser are certificates of authenticity, which some companies will provide. (The value of working with a knowledgeable and reputable dealer becomes clear here.)

- Realize that some scents do not exist in any form other than synthetic. There is nothing wrong with enjoying a replicated plant aroma if you keep in mind that it is not viable for clinical aromatherapy. Such scents include amber, apple, cucumber, gardenia, coconut, lily of the valley, lilac, musk, and strawberry.

- Remember that some essences can be extracted only by using solvents. The resulting products are not essential oils but rather absolutes, concretes, enfleurages, and oleoresins. Examples include oakmoss, tuberose, vanilla, and violet leaf.

- You can recognize absolutes, such as jasmine or violet leaf, by their small quantities (measured in drams or grams) and high prices.

- Some essences may be obtained through both solvent means (in which case they are absolutes) and steam distillation (in which case they are essential oils). Rose is a good example: The essential oil is referred to as "rose attar" or "otto" and will take on a crystallized or gel-like appearance when chilled; the absolute rose will not.

- If a company makes available "lotting" numbers or "batching" dates, pay attention. A batching date tells you when your oil was bottled by your supplier. If you have a lot number (when your essential oil was distilled), you can often repurchase from the same lot and thus retain consistency of odor and other characteristics.

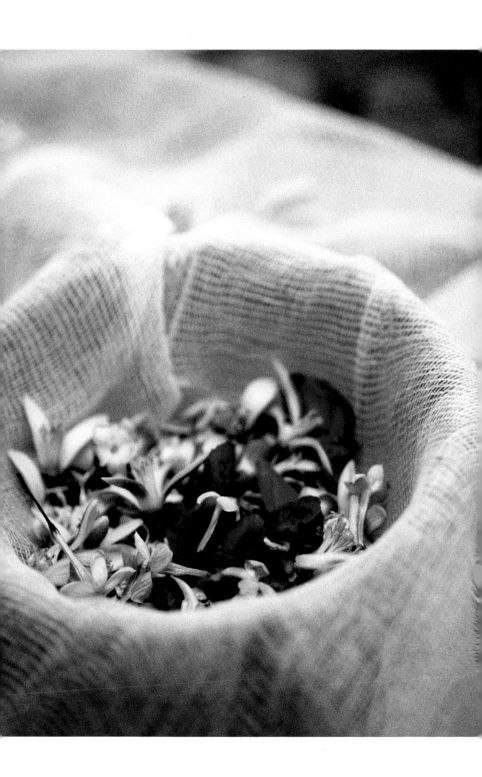

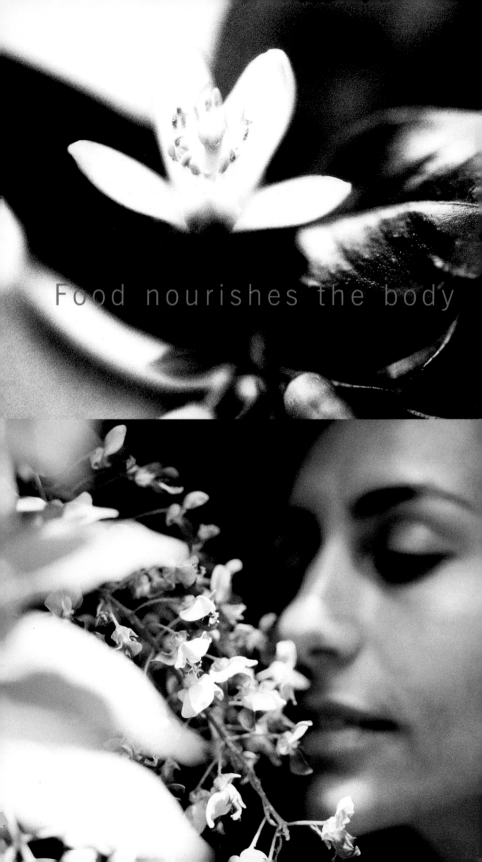

Food nourishes the body

safETY

When choosing to work with essential oils for therapeutic results, rather
than purely as an enhancement in aroma, it is best to seek the counsel
and guidance of a trained professional aromatherapist or aromatologist.
Thus, you will be less likely to choose essential oils that in long-term
usage or improper application could be potentially harmful or create
skin sensitivities. The essential oils chosen for this book are generally
considered acceptable for beginning aromatherapy. The reader is

ut flowers nourish the soul.
—Ancient Proverb

encouraged to familiarize yourself with literature that supports both
the safety and efficacy of aromatherapy and to take note of the specific
safeties mentioned in the basic (pages 89–99) and sensuous (pages
101–113) cupboards of this book.

Take special care when choosing essential oils for children,
pregnant women, frail individuals, and the elderly. Most essential
oils are too strong for children under the age of five. Stick to the very
safest oils, such as lavender, chamomile, lemon, geranium, rose attar,
pure neroli, and tangerine. Always dilute the essential oil using 1 to 2
teaspoons of a carrier, such as a vegetal oil, nut oil, seed oil, or fatty
milk, to 1 to 3 drops of the chosen essential oil. When preparing an
aromatic bath, make sure to thoroughly agitate the water to disperse
the essences.

The use of certain essential oils is not advised in the presence
of some physical conditions. These conditions include (but are not
limited to) pregnancy, breast-feeding, hormonal disturbances
(such as estrogenic cancer), photosensitivity, dermal sensitization,
hypotensive and hypertensive imbalances, liver or kidney disease or

imbalance, asthma, diabetes, epilepsy, and anorexia. Many oils should not be used with anticoagulants and can interfere with other health supplements, such as iodine and iron.

general children's dose reductions

age	dose
5 to 8 years old	1/6 to 1/3 adult dose
8 to 12 years old	1/3 to 1/2 adult dose
12 to 15 years old	1/2 to 2/3 adult dose

Essential oils are highly concentrated. Always research the recommended dosage. Remember, with essential oils more is not necessarily better. Larger doses may negate the possible therapeutic effect of a recommended dose and may even be toxic.

Essential oils tend to accumulate in the body. For this reason, each week it is advisable to take a break from using a particular oil over a 24- to 48-hour period. If you are using an oil frequently, drink extra water to aid in eliminating toxins, and if you choose not to take breaks, restrict yourself to mild oils and reduce the amounts you use.

Indications of allergy or mild sensitivity to essential oils may include slight skin rashes or sensitivity, mild headache or dizziness, nausea, and mucous membrane irritation. It is important that the reader understand that essential oils need to be not merely treated as a pretty aroma, but respected for their phyto-pharmacology potentials. More dramatic indications are usually experienced as a result of improper or overuse of essential oils. If any abnormal conditions follow the use of essential oils, discontinue using them immediately and consult your physician.

If you are using homeopathic remedies, it is best to check with your physician before using essential oils. Many oils, such as black pepper, eucalyptus, and peppermint, are thought to counteract homeopathic therapy.

As with other medications, keep essential oils out of the reach of children. Never take essential oils internally on your own initiative. If you or another person swallows an essential oil, call your local poison control center immediately. Do not induce vomiting or give water if breathing or swallowing is difficult.

Keep essential oils away from the eyes and mucous membranes. If an essential oil gets into the eye, do not rub it. Saturate a cotton ball with whole milk or vegetal oil and pat gently over the area affected and over the closed eyelid. In instances of severe irritation, flood the eye area with lukewarm water for a full 15 minutes.

As a general rule you should dilute oils before applying them to the skin. Some essential oils are regarded as safe to use "neat," or undiluted, but never apply more than 3 drops of undiluted essential oil to your skin. A skin patch test is advised whether essential oils are to be applied diluted or undiluted.

SKIN PATCH TEST

Begin by washing and thoroughly drying the area on which you will be testing your essential oil. To test a pure essential oil or blend of oils, place a single drop in the crook of your arm. Bend your elbow, grasping your shoulder with your hand, and wait three to five minutes. If there is any stinging, swab the area with a cotton ball saturated with milk or vegetal oil, then wash the area thoroughly with soap and water.

To test a prepared massage lotion or oil, apply a small amount to the forearm. Cover with a small piece of gauze or cotton, secured with adhesive tape. Leave for 24 hours unless irritation is noticeable before, in which case wipe a cotton ball dipped in whole milk or vegetal oil over the area. Then thoroughly wash the area with soap and water.

storage

Heat, light, and air all detract from the therapeutic powers of an essential oil. Store your essential oils and prepared formulas in a cool, dark place and make sure the tops of the bottles or vials are firmly secured. Even when working with your oils, as in blending, keep them capped when they are not in use. Use pharmaceutical glass bottles and vials made of integrated-color glass to shade the contents from light. The vials are available in emerald green, bromo or cobalt blue, violet, and amber. Plastic bottles may deteriorate and damage the oils. When correctly stored, many distilled essential oils will keep up to a year, and many can even mature aromatically with time.

An essential oil will begin to develop a cloudy appearance as it begins to oxidize. You may choose to replace the air in larger containers of essential oils with an inert gas such as nitrogen (which you can find at premium wine stores); this helps prevent oxidation.

Never store your oils with the dropper inside the bottle. Keep the dropper separate and protected. Clean after each session of use with 100 percent grain alcohol, denatured alcohol, or good-quality vodka.

Essential oils are flammable materials and should be stored in a well-ventilated area away from heat sources. An essential oil can act as a solvent and may damage polished wood or enameled, veneered, and synthetic surfaces.

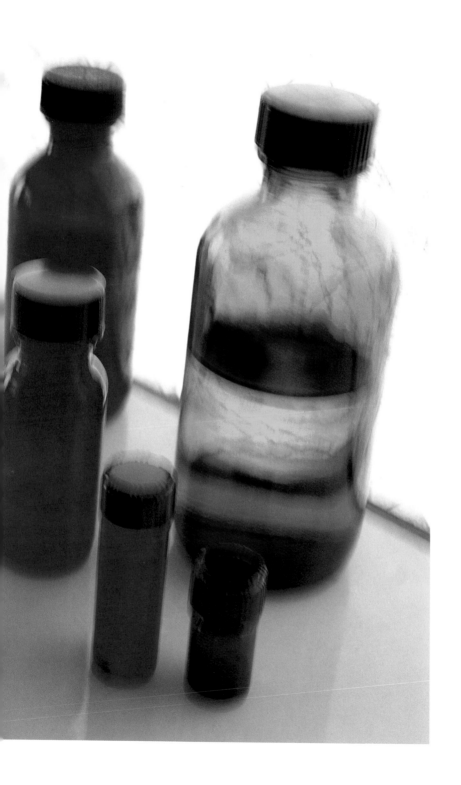

And in the moment
betwixt the breathing in
and the breathing out

is hidden all the mysteries
of the Infinite Garden.

—Edmond Bordeaux Szekely

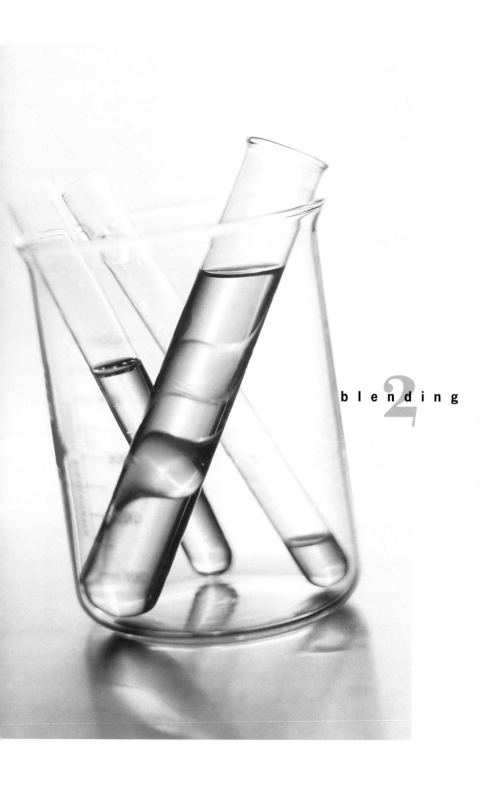

blending **2**

Have you ever stopped to delight in your sense

of smell, to wonder at the variety of different scents that can be

enjoyed in but one of the tens of thousands of breaths you take daily?

A simple walk in the garden can include the aromas of breeze, rain,

mist, earth, stone, moss, grass, leaves, bark, flowers, and fauna. It is

often difficult to find the words to describe aromatic essences. But if

we take the time, we discover that each essential oil has its own

unique personality. Its traits include its color, its texture or "feel,"

its mobility or viscosity, its taste, and its aroma.

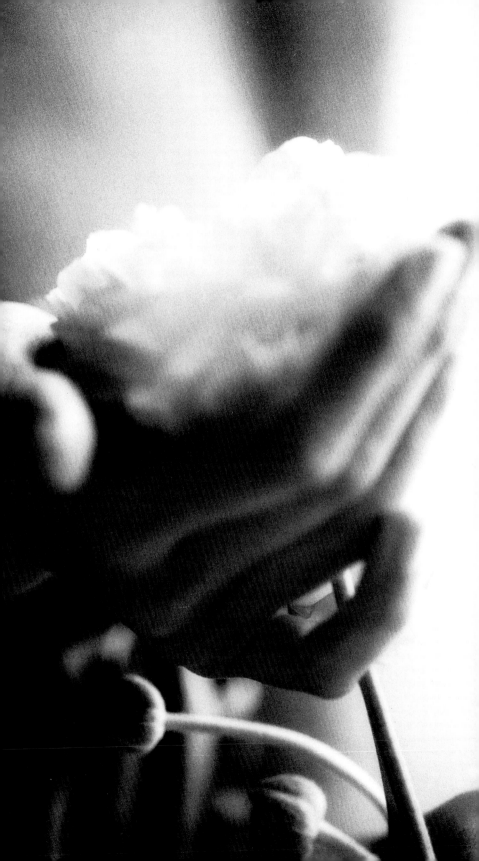

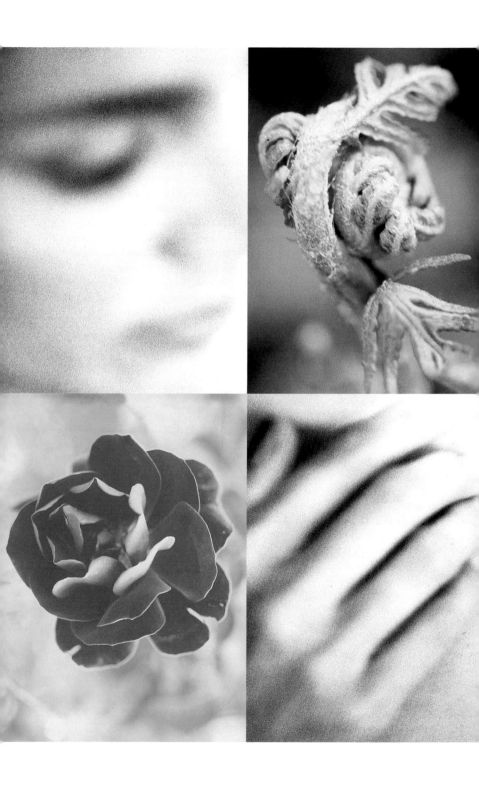

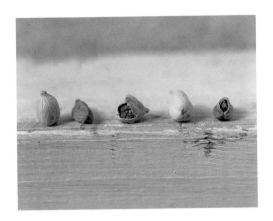

THE LANGUAGE OF SCENT

Like fine wine, aromatic essences, or essential oils, require a language all their own. We can talk of their classifications, identifying the scents, or aromas, they remind us of; we can try to pinpoint their characteristics, describing the sensation the odor creates in us; or we can define their "notes," a term from perfumery describing the immediacy of an odor and its rate of evaporation. "Tones" is another term sometimes colloquially used instead of "notes." When you become familiar with these aromatic distinctions, you can begin to combine essential oils in the orchestration known as blending.

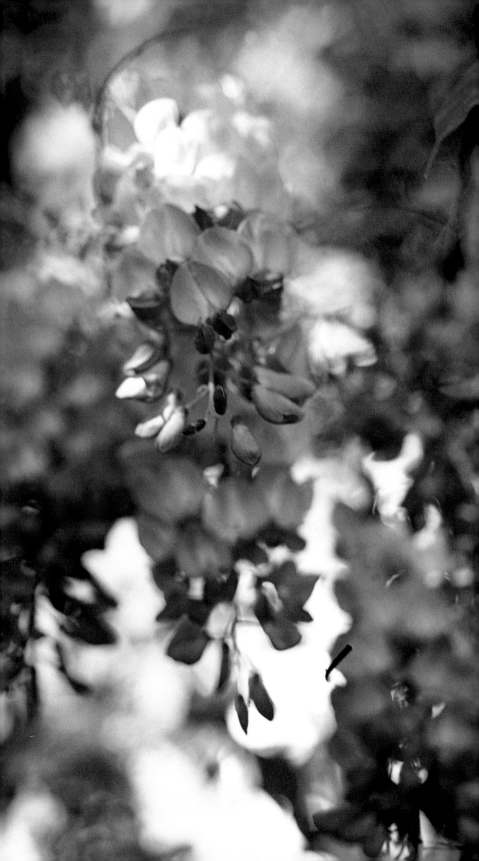

classifications

ANIMALIC (aka CAPRILIC):
This term recalls the ancient use of
animal secretions and by-products
such as musk, civet, and ambergris.
Today aromatherapy does not adhere
to the use of these products, even
though many cultures still incorporate
their use. Still, some essences, such
as ambrette and spikenard, are said
to have the distinctive attribute of
animalic.

ANISIC: Derived from anise, this
term describes a licorice quality. Anisic
scents tend to be sweet like sugar.
Essences that typify an anisic scent
are fennel and basil.

BALSAMIC: Just as balsam has a
resinous quality, a balsamic scent has
an oily, sweet, resinous nature that
can range from a sweetened glue to
a caramelized root beer. Essences
that typify this scent are peru balsam,
benzoin, and the heart of juniper.

BURNT: This term refers to an
"overdone" quality. Often vetiver,
which is referred to in this manner,
is "burned" in distillation. If done
properly, a superior scent will emerge
with a distinctive green, grassy note.
Some refer to this as an "empyrean"
note, linked to what the ancients
believed to be the purest element, fire.

CAMPHORACEOUS: This is
the scent that "bites." It jumps up
your nose and often causes a sneeze.
It has a medicinal quality to it that
resembles camphor. The scent of oils
rich in 1.8 cineole, such as eucalyptus
and rosemary, is often described as
camphoraceous.

CITRUS: This refers to a fresh,
tangy, sweet quality that can range
from a light crispness to a pithy
warmth. Lemon, lime, and bergamot
typify this scent.

CONIFER: This scent elicits the sense of deep breathing that evergreens coax from us. Conifer oils smell refreshingly green, with characteristics of leaf, cone, and bark in their resinous base tones. Fir, pine, and spruce typify this scent, and juniper shares this tone.

EARTHY: Think of drenching rain on a parched earth. When the rain stops, one can smell the clays and moss whose scents lay dormant without the enticement of moisture. Patchouli, vetiver, and oakmoss typify this aromatic quality.

FECAL: Essences as beautiful as jasmine and tuberose are rewarded with this seemingly unlikely description. The indole-rich scent of these oils expresses the rich bounty of life at their core.

FLORAL: This general odor classification describes the category where flowers reign supreme. Here we find the champa and the rose, among others.

FRUITY: These are the jubilant scents: robust, juicy, splashy, plump, vivacious. One immediately envisions a ripened orange. However, "fruity" oftentimes applies to a flowering herb such as chamomile, which exhibits an "apple note," or black pepper, which displays a "plump" attitude.

GREEN: To get a sense of this aromatic distinction, take three leaves from three different plant species. Crush each individually between your fingers and smell. The underlying aroma is similar, is it not? The moist, fresh, and clear scent gives one the impression of the color green. Multifolded helichrysum and violet leaf typify this scent.

HERBACEOUS: When an herb begins to fade, it emits a green, pungent, vegetative, woodlike scent. Typifying this herbaceous quality are lavender, marjoram, hyssop, chamomile, and many others.

METALLIC: This term describes a scent like that of stainless steel rinsed with cool water. Peppermint and fir have a metallic tone.

MINTY: This tone, which draws its name from the family of mints, captures one quality in particular, that of menthol. It is sharp and tart and goes right up your nose and retreats behind your eyes. Often it evens out to a warm, green tanginess. Here we find spearmint and peppermint.

MOSSY: Think of the moist, warm, shadowed depths of the forest, where the mosses relish existence. Essences supreme in this quality are oakmoss and violet leaf.

OILY: This describes a "fatty" quality, easily understood when one recalls the scent of carrier oils used in massage, such as almond and olive. Many essences, such as ylang ylang, display a rotund, fatty quality as well.

PEPPERY OR PEPPERED: Related to the black peppercorn, the pepper tree's dried fruit, this term applies to a dry and woody scent with a spicy heat.

ROSACEOUS: This describes a heady, cheerful, and optimistic odor, like that of a rose. Rose damask and cabbage, geranium, and palmarosa typify this scent.

SPICY: Experiencing a spicy scent is like riding the escalator into the center of a pepper or a rhizome. Just as with food, spicy to one person may not be spicy to another, but a spicy tone is usually imbued with a sensation of heat and a glorious pungency, such as as with cloves and cinnamon

WOODY: Many essences, particularly those that incorporate stalks and twigs, display this quality. There is a subtle richness weighted by dryness with immense staying power. Essences that typify this tone are sandalwood and cedarwood.

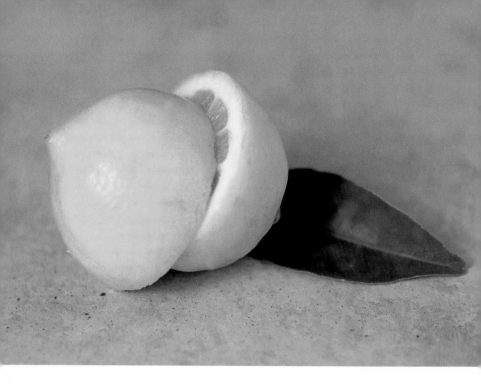

characteristics

BALANCED: An essence—orange is an example—that displays no struggle. No component outshines the others.

DIFFUSIVE: An essence that permeates the atmosphere and the senses as soon as the cap is removed. Geranium typifies this description.

DISTINCTIVE: An essence, like violet leaf, that has a pronounced individuality.

DRY: An essence that reminds one of the desert. Most essences described as dry are labeled "powdered" when they are nearly evaporated. Patchouli is characterized as dry.

EFFERVESCENT: An essence that is scintillating, like a sparkling soda. A good example is yuzu.

FLAT: An essence that lacks a robust personality or layering in its temperament. This term is clearly apparent in a resinoid, such as balsam peru or styrax benzoin, which has been exposed to air over a period of time.

POWDERED: An essence, such as violet leaf, with a hint of softness, like baby powder.

FRESH: An essence that promotes liveliness and joy and evokes a feeling of cleanliness. Lemon essential oil typically has a fresh character.

RICH: An essence of ardor and overwhelming sumptuousness. Rose is typically rich.

HARSH: An essence exhibiting a primitive nature; unpolished; unrefined. Lemongrass in a crude distillation can be harsh, although when properly produced, lemongrass essential oil is refreshing and lightly green, like fresh grass.

SHARP: An essence that is biting and intrusive. Tea tree, for example, exhibits a sharp character.

SMOOTH: An essence that seems endless. Sandalwood and melissa often reflect this quality.

HEAVY: An essence of profound weight and depth, like ylang ylang.

SMOKY: An essence that brings to mind hickory chips and campfires at dusk: the heart of cypress and vetiver.

LIGHT: An essence of delicacy and high volatility, such as neroli.

MULTIFACETED: An essence that seems to display no boundaries as layer upon layer unfolds. Helichrysum produces this experience.

SWEET: An essence exhibiting a hint of nectar, a confectionary of the botanical realm. Anise and bay laurel can be characterized as sweet.

WARM: An essence that displays sultry enthusiasm or passion, such as rose or ginger.

MUSTY: An essence reeking of the catacombs of a library—vetiver, for one.

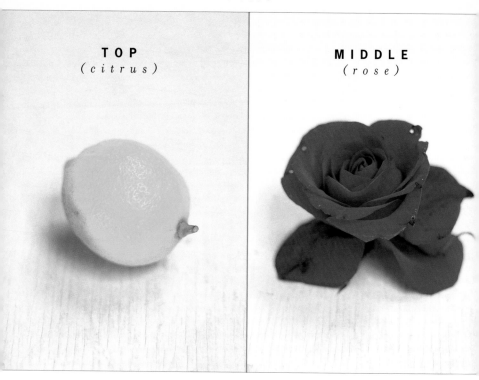

TOP
(*c i t r u s*)

MIDDLE
(*r o s e*)

Borrowing from the language of music, we define the aromatic levels of a fragrant essence in notes. Notes are the impressions left by the essence and are based on its evaporation rate and how intensely the essence affects the nose. The basic note categories are top, middle, and base. Opinions can differ on which oils are characterized by which note. Many oils are capable of bridging the octaves between top and middle, middle and base.

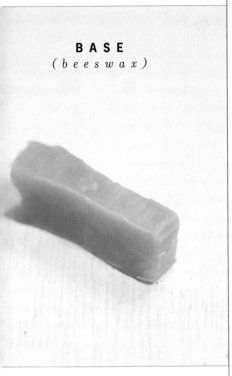

BASE
(b e e s w a x)

TOP NOTES: Top notes, also referred to as *notes de tête*, are the first to connect with your nose and usually make the most powerful impression. They are the hardest notes to synthetically reproduce. Top notes are light, sharply scintillating, piercing, and tangy in tone. They "top off" a blend, comprising about 25 to 40 percent, and their impressions remain for about 30 minutes. Just as quickly as they burst aggressively forward, they retreat and evaporate. Many top notes have a transforming effect on emotional malaise as they soar and uplift and attach themselves quickly and succinctly. If notes were the instruments in a symphony orchestra, top notes would be the flutes and violins.

Top notes include eucalyptus, lemon, mandarin, peppermint, rosemary, and tea tree. Oils that bridge the octave from top notes to middle notes include black pepper, cardamom, lavender, linden, mandarin, neroli, peppermint, and rosemary.

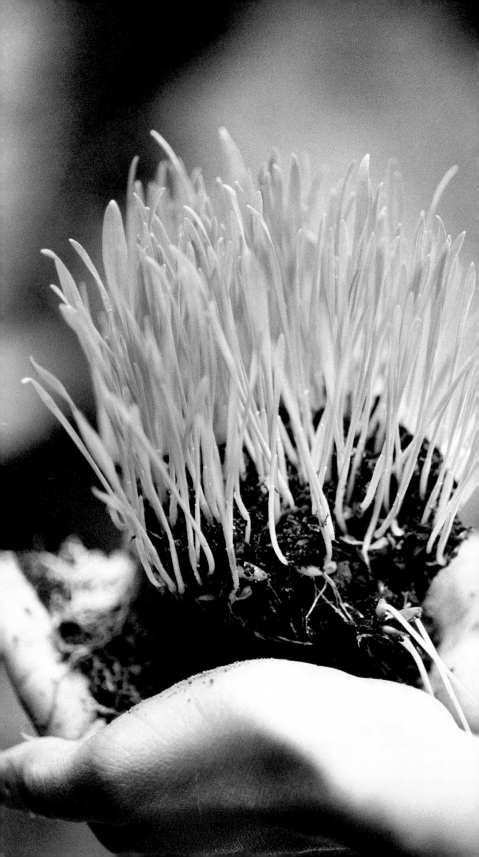

MIDDLE NOTES: These are the oils that are rich, heady, robust, and warm in character. Middle notes modify a blend and are the easiest to reproduce synthetically. Within a single essence, they are the least characteristic notes, but in a synergy they become the body, the heat, the bouquet. They are often referred to as *notes de coeur*. Middle notes are detected usually after about half an hour. They can be discerned directly beneath the top notes, making their strongest appearance after one to three hours and often holding true for one to two days. These are the essences that make up the bulk— about 50 to 70 percent—of a blend. These are the "fine wine" notes. They mature as they age and often improve as they are opened and subjected to air. These are the notes that create balance and unite the mind, body, and spirit. In an orchestra, these would be the clarinets, the cellos.

Middle notes include black pepper, cardamom, roman chamomile, clary sage, geranium, lavender, and linden. Oils that bridge the octave from middle notes to base notes include frankincense, ginger, jasmine, rose, vanilla, and violet leaf.

BASE NOTES: Essential oils with distinctive base notes, or *notes de fond*, include cedarwood, jasmine, sandalwood, vanilla, vetiver, and ylang ylang. These notes surface in one to five hours and can easily last up to 24 hours with clarified evenness. In a blend it is best to limit them to about 5 to 10 percent. They are the heaviest notes and offer sensuous depth, strength, virility, and resonance. These notes are referred to as a synergy's flavoring and fixative, since they hold a blend together and give it staying power. These notes possess a sedating quality and can be used as such in a therapeutic blend. They are the last notes to fade (or dry out) and they are often the most adulterated of the notes. In an orchestra these would be the bassoons or the kettle drums.

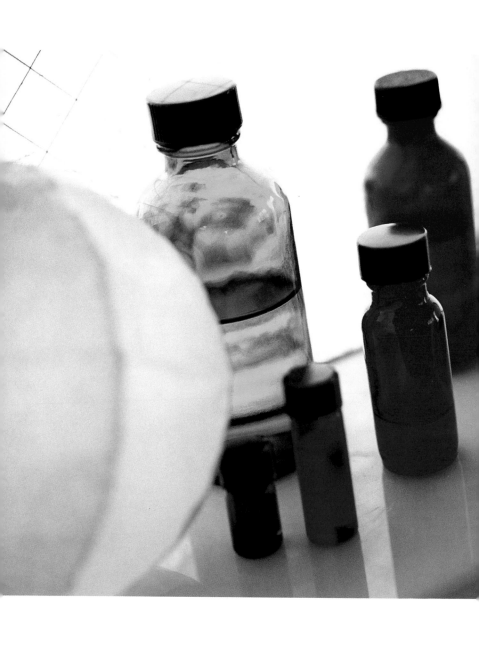

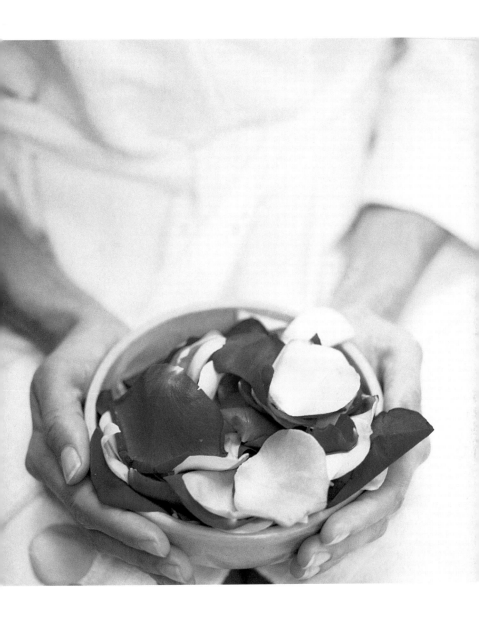

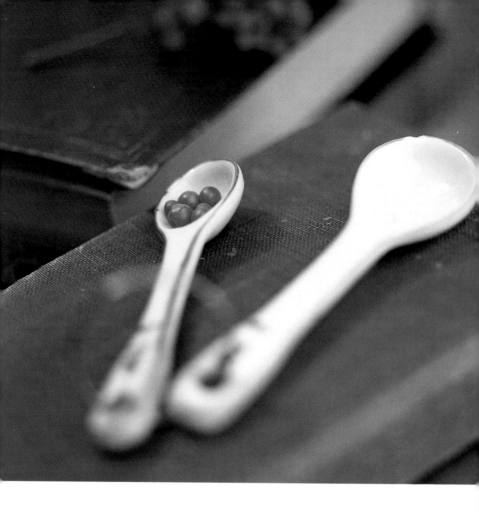

Preparing to Blend

A balanced and aromatically pleasing blend of oils (or "synergy")
is one in which the components complement each other through both
their therapeutic actions and their aromatic structuring. Mixing
oils with similar properties will accentuate and magnify those
qualities. For example, a lavender and mandarin blend will soothe,
balance, nurture, and relax. Rosemary and grapefruit will invigorate,
challenge, and strengthen. Vetiver and patchouli will stimulate the
senses and encourage physical stamina and centering.

At the hands of a skilled blender and aromatherapist, synergies become complex vehicles to support health and heighten pleasure, with different therapeutic actions and aromatic characteristics working together to create a multilayered effect. For instance a synergy created for severe musculoskeletal pain, such as with arthritis, can be complemented with oils that will reduce the pain, spasm, and inflammation. They are able to warm the tissue area, acting as a rubefacient and vasodilator, while they also address the emotional stresses and strains, such as depression, anxiety, or the inability to concentrate, that are caused by the unrelenting pain.

The aromatic appeal of the fragrant essential oils should always be of primary importance. Even when essential oils are used for health purposes, there are no essences that cannot be combined so that the outcome is aromatically pleasant as well as therapeutic. These are the elements to consider when you begin blending aromatic essences and unleash their fragrant vapors.

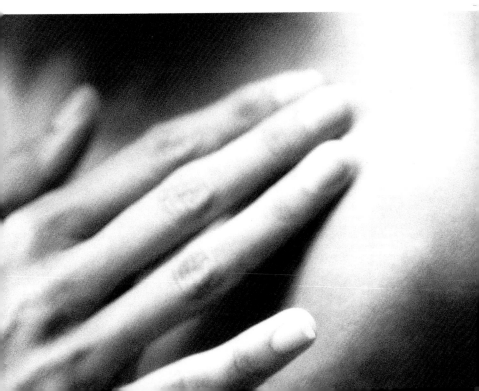

composing a blend

Limit your first aromatic blends to three to six essential oils. Not only will this help you avoid costly errors, but it will let you experience the relationship of oils in a blend. As you build strong relationships with your essences, your synergies also will develop in their complexities.

When planning a synergy, work outward from the core of the blend. Warm, spicy notes such as black pepper, cardamom, coriander, and ginger work well at the center, as does a hearty, minty floral such as geranium, an herbaceously pungent and earthy chamomile, or a green conifer such as cypress or juniper. Lilting, tangy, sweet essential oils such as grapefruit, lemon, mandarin, and sweet orange offer an excellent topping to a synergy. Your base note might rely on the resinous, balsamic wood tones of sandalwood, a musty, "smoked" root such as a vetiver, or a heady floral such as rose or ylang ylang. In a good oil blend, the components dance in complement to each other's refrain. Sharp, tangy, sweet oils such as lemon, lime, grapefruit, and mandarin love the warm spices of black pepper, cardamom, coriander, and ginger. Soft, balsamic wood tones such as cedarwood and sandalwood wonderfully complement the florals of geranium, rose, or ylang ylang. Bergamot does an amazing chameleon's dance between the layers of a well-defined synergy.

You will note that many aromatic essences not only bridge the notes within a blend but also have the ability to move and adapt within a blend, going from a top range all the way to a base note if complemented with the right essences. Good examples are the spiciness of cardamom and ginger, the floral herbaceousness of lavender, and the robust fruitiness of bergamot.

A skilled blender will also pay attention to the differences in aromatic tone created through regional characteristics of the essences.

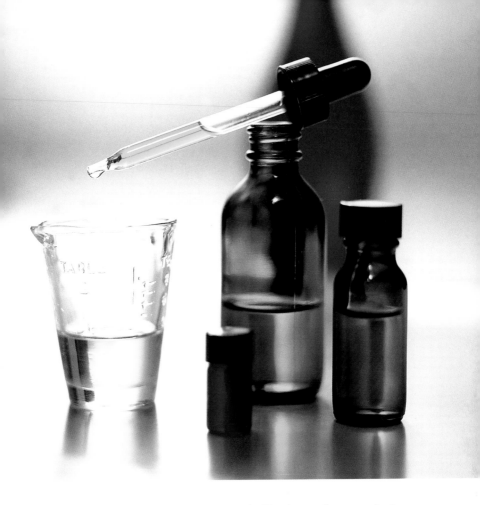

A lavender from the shores of the Pacific Northwest, for example, has a very different tonal quality from one from the fields of Provence. A lemon oil from Florida barely compares in strength, warmth, and complexity to one from Italy. The differing chemistry of oils also has an effect on their therapeutic efficacy.

Before you dive into blending, take a moment to analyze the synergy you are hoping to develop. Aromatic dynamics that sound brilliant on paper may prove quite unpleasant once blended. Or when applied to your skin, your blend may take on a completely different character than it displayed in its blending receptacle. A few precautions can avert a costly aromatic disaster.

● A S K   Y O U R S E L F , What is the intention of this synergy? Is its purpose purely aromatic or are you seeking a specific thera- peutic support? Always research your essential oils' chemistry and therapeutic actions well. Consider all safety precautions when making your choices for your blends. When in doubt, stick to oils regarded as generally safe and nontoxic. For therapeutic synergies make sure to work with the purest grade essential oils possible. And always remember that your blend will provoke an emotional response upon inhalation.

● A P P L Y   1   O R   2   D R O P S of each essential oil to be used on a professional test strip, damp cotton ball, or unbleached blot- ting paper. Allow them a moment of vaporization. If the resulting scent is not pleasing, waste of the oils is minimal.

● T E S T   Y O U R   B L E N D by adding 5 to 8 drops of your synergy to 1 to 2 teaspoons of unscented carrier oil (such as jojoba). Apply to the inside of your wrist and the top of your hand or arm. This will allow the scent to merge with your skin's chem- istry. You will be able to see how the aromatic notes break away, as well as judge the staying power of your synergy. You will also be able to detect any possible skin reaction. If possible, apply the same test to anyone you will be working with.

● K E E P   I N   M I N D that a synergy, especially for use as a fragrance, is best after a maturation period of a week to 10 days. If time permits, put your synergy aside to see how your essences come together in union. If any of your synergies prove displeas- ing, use them around sink drains, or add to suds and water to clean areas such as garbage pails, pet areas, tiles, and flooring. Try not to waste these precious aromatics.

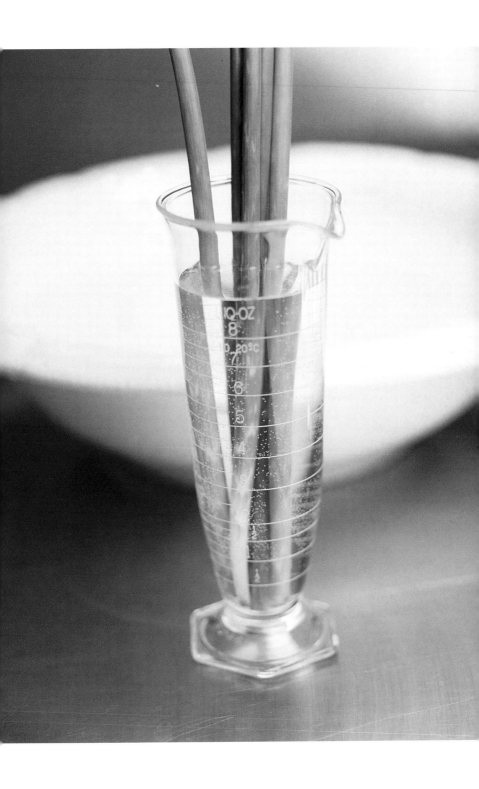

A few technical notes before you start: Work space is vitally important. Temperatures need to be moderate, and the room should be well ventilated. Have fresh water close at hand and sip it while working, especially if you are working with your essences for long periods of time, which blending may require. Keep a white cotton washcloth or T-shirt nearby to breathe into periodically to clear your nasal pathways. Give your nose a break between odors by inhaling the aroma of fresh organic coffee beans. Drinking lemon-infused water can also help flush odor residues.

Keep your droppers clean between uses. Store them in 15 milliliter amber dropper bottles filled with grain alcohol or vodka. Label the bottles "top," "middle," and "base"; when you are blending, use the dropper that corresponds to the note of the oil you are working with, flushing it with alcohol between uses. Refill the bottles with fresh alcohol every week, dispensing of old alcohol into drains to deodorize them. Take care of your blending surfaces; spills of essences may result in damage to varnished wood and synthetic surfaces. Tiled counters are best.

Francis Thompson wrote, "One cannot pluck a flower without troubling a star." Those words always catch me unaware each spring just as I am tempted to bend and pluck one of the first blooms rising from the remnants of the winter's mulch. To me, they express how our planet must quake each time her natural bounty is plucked or, worse, discarded. When you begin your aromatic blending, think of how precious the bounty of your small vial is, how many pounds of botanic material were needed to obtain your liquid gold, and how much time and effort went into its cultivation, harvest, and extraction. With those thoughts in mind, you embark on a journey not only of pleasure and purpose but that takes on a sense of the divine.

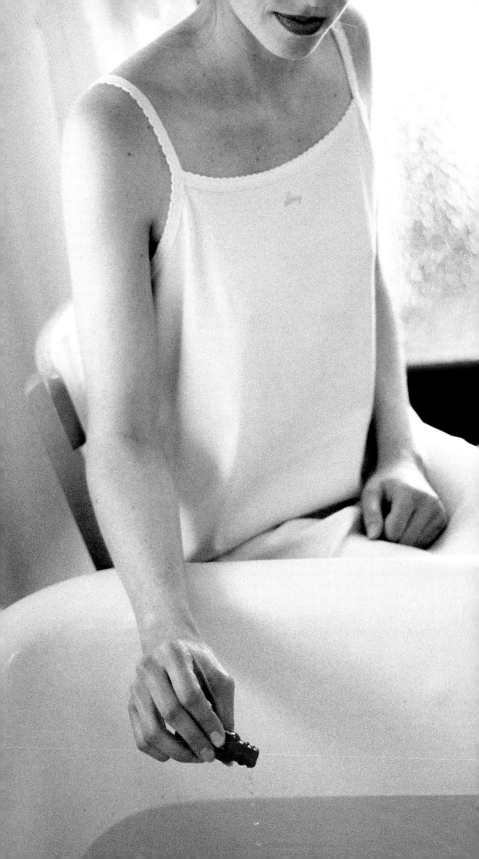

Believe nothing, no matter where you read
said it, unless it agrees with your own

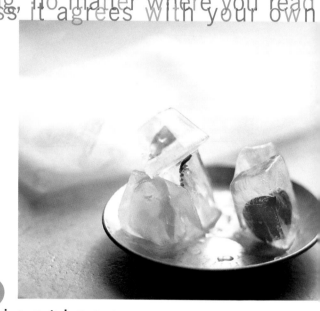

3 **applications**

it or who has said it, not even if I have

reason and your own common sense.

—Gautama Buddha

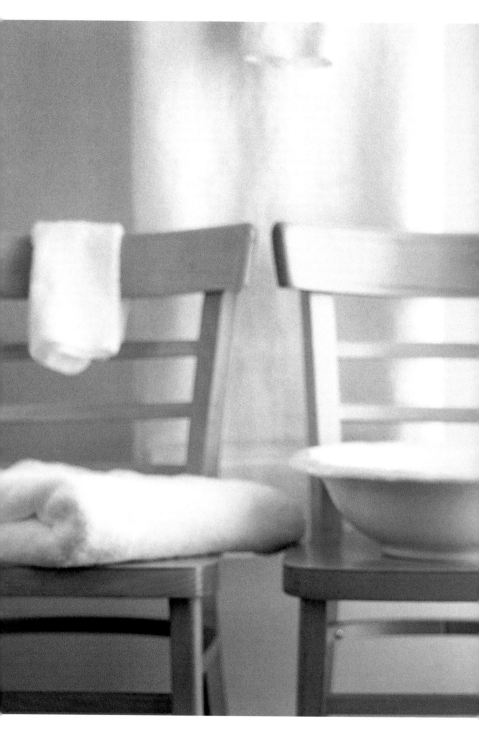

For ages, aromatic essences have been used for healing and for pleasure. Today the widespread production and sale of essential oils makes it easy for us to continue the tradition by adding essences to the air we breathe and the products we use. This chapter describes some of the most common ways to incorporate aromatic essences into your daily life. I have included some of my own favorite synergies and recipes.

Inhalation

Inhalation is one of the simplest ways to enjoy the aroma and rejuvenating power of essential oils. It also offers the fastest form of absorption into the body. When you inhale a scent, it triggers a neurochemical response in the brain, it infiltrates the small air sacs in the lungs, and it is passed almost immediately into the bloodstream. If you are pregnant or have asthma, epilepsy, or other health problems, check with your primary care physician before using essential oils in this manner (see pages 29–32).

direct inhalation

Mix the following recipes in small vials and dispense as directed.

Direct inhalation can provide the perfect antidote for a headache, stress, or anxiety. Simply uncork a vial and breathe in. Or sprinkle 2 or 3 drops of a single oil or of a synergy of oils onto an unscented tissue or cotton ball, hold it under your nose, and inhale. The cotton ball can be dropped into a plastic bag to be inhaled when needed or can be tucked into your pillowcase at night.

THE SOUL'S REPOSE

7 drops sweet orange
  or red mandarin
2 drops violet leaf
2 drops sandalwood
1 drop rose attar

palm inhalation

This is my "essential" application—another form of direct inhalation. It is a perfect method for centering yourself and clearing your mind of distractions. Place no more than 3 drops of an oil or a synergy of oils into the palm of your hand, vigorously rub to warm the oil, cup your hands to your nose, and breathe deeply three times.

CLARITY

11 drops grapefruit
9 drops lemon
6 drops peppermint
5 drops basil
3 drops black pepper
2 drops marjoram

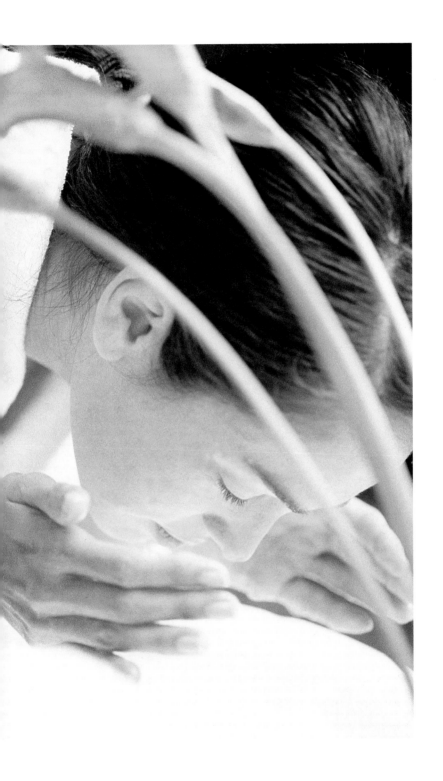

steam inhalation

BODY'S DEFENSE

5 drops lemon

4 drops pine

(*Pinus sylvestris*)

3 drops eucalyptus

2 drops ginger

2 drops cardamom

This method is especially beneficial for sinus complaints, influenza, colds, and coughs but should be avoided if you have asthma. The steam carries the essential oils quickly to the bronchial area, affording a soothing yet forceful decongestant. Add 4 to 7 drops of a synergy to a bowl of boiling water. Cover both your head and the bowl with a tented towel and inhale for five to 10 minutes. For young children, omit the towel and just allow the vapors to rise around the head.

diffusion

SOLAR REFRAIN

6 drops red mandarin

4 drops lemon

3 drops clary sage

2 drops chamomile

2 drops geranium

1 drop nutmeg

To refresh, invigorate, calm, and warm your emotions and spirit, the diffusion of aromatic essences is an absolute must! Stores today are filled with tiny vessels used as heated diffusers, such as aromatic lamps, clay pots, and light bulb rings. Use these diffusers as directed by the instructions that accompany the product. Electric, cool air diffusion methods are those most widely used by aromatherapists as a therapeutic tool. Not only do they add aroma to a room, but they can clear the air of germs and bacteria. To use a professional diffuser, add 20 to 30 drops of a synergy to the receptacle and run it for 15 to 30 minutes, three times a day.

compresses

Compresses are a wonderful way to relieve arthritis, sprains, and general aches and pains. There are two primary methods of compressing: cold and hot. For each, pour approximately two cups of water into a clean stainless steel or porcelain bowl and add 4 to 6 drops of a synergy. Agitate the water to disperse the oil, then dip cotton gauze or a cloth into the water, wring it out, and apply it to the afflicted area. Repeat the application several times over a period of 15 minutes, keeping the temperature of the compress constant.

cold compresses

HEADEASE

5 drops lemon

5 drops peppermint

3 drops lavender

Instant cold compresses can be kept handy by infusing ice cubes and storing them in your freezer. Add 1 or 2 drops of an individual oil or a synergy to each compartment of an ice tray filled with water, and use the frozen cubes to relieve pain, inflammation, or sunburn.

hot compresses

STRETCHING

THE LIMITS

5 drops rosemary

5 drops red mandarin

4 drops chamomile

3 drops jasmine
  samboc

2 drops ginger

Hot compresses enable a much faster penetration of essential oils. They work well to treat menstrual pain, constipation, and tooth and muscle aches. Draw the water as hot as you can tolerate it, but less hot when applying a compress to the facial area. Water that is too hot may break fragile capillaries. To maintain the heat of a compress, cover it with plastic wrap.

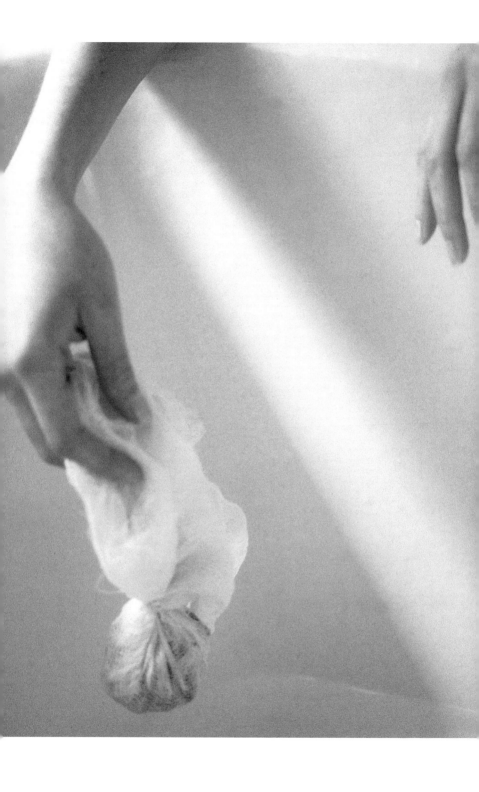

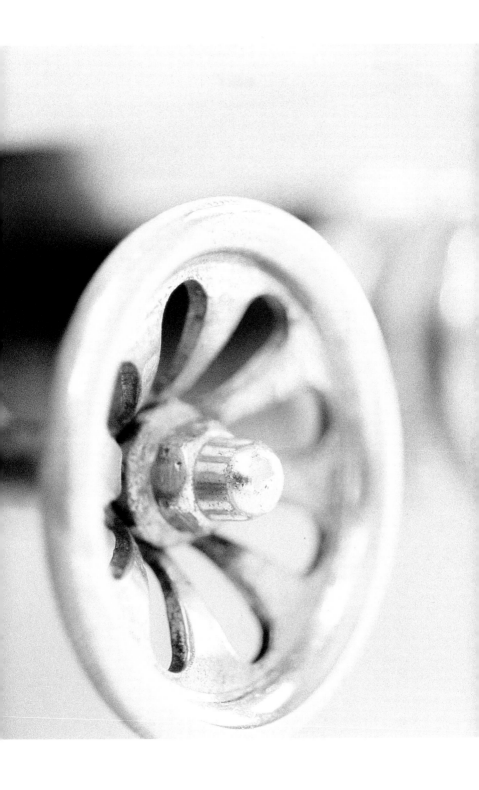

DRY BRUSHING

To enhance detoxification, stimulate circulation, and restore vigor, dry brushing is a must. It's also the perfect exfoliation preparation before an aromatic bath or shower. Apply 1 or 2 drops of essential oil or a synergy of oils to a clean natural bristle brush. Always begin at your feet, lightly brushing the skin in a clockwise, circular motion upward toward your heart. From the bottoms of the feet, move to the tops and work your way up your legs and over your buttocks. Next, brush both sides of your hands, then move up your arms to your elbows, forearms, and shoulders. Gently and rhythmically brush your abdomen and torso. Women can brush the upper chest and back but should avoid the breast area.

JUMP START

6 drops grapefruit

5 drops cypress

4 drops lemon

3 drops rosemary

2 drops cardamom

2 drops geranium

2 drops black pepper

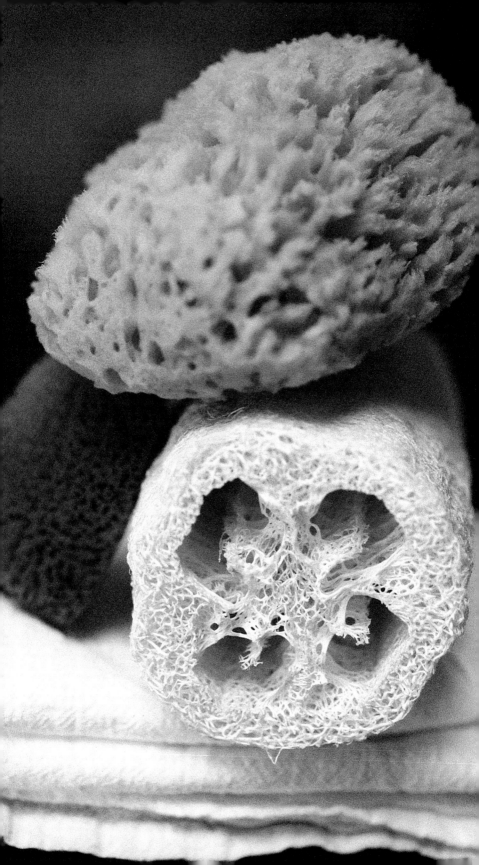

three simple bath recipes

SIMPLE BATH OR SHOWER GEL

To 4 ounces of good-quality unscented foaming bath or shower gel, add a mixture of 25 to 35 drops of essential oils. Add 2 to 3 tablespoons to your bath water or squeeze onto your loofah or sponge.

SIMPLE BATH OIL

Pour 4 ounces of a carrier oil into a jar. In another lidded jar, combine 30 to 50 drops of a synergy of essential oils and 1 teaspoon of simple tincture benzoin, and shake it vigorously. Add this mixture to the carrier oil and shake again. Use 2 tablespoons per bath.

SIMPLE BATH SALTS

Place 1 cup of sea, mineral, or Epsom salt (or combination of all three, equaling 1 cup) in a lidded container. Add 1/4 cup of baking soda to reduce clumping. Then add 10 to 20 drops of essential oil and shake vigorously. Add half of this mixture to your bath.

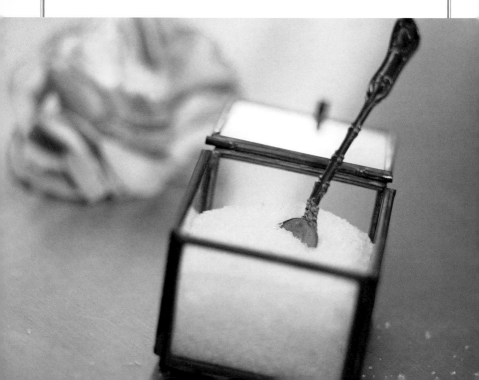

Bathing is truly one of the most enjoyable means of administering essential oils. The ancient Greek word meaning "to bathe" also means "to drive sadness from the mind." An aromatic bath can either relax a tense body or stimulate a fatigued body.

In a warm bath, essential oils are absorbed in two ways: through the skin (pores, hair follicles, and blood vessels) and through the nasal passages as the essences waft to your nose. It is safest to dilute your oils in prepared salts, oils, and soaps before adding them to bath water, but 3 to 5 drops of an individual essential oil or 10 to 15 drops of a synergy may be added directly to your bathwater if you are careful to disperse the oil thoroughly by agitating the water before entering your tub. For maximum therapeutic effect, soak for at least 10 to 15 minutes. Keep in mind that bathing need not be a full-body bath. An aromatic shower can be nearly as effective. Create and aromatic shower gel by infusing a good body soap with your essences—5 or 6 drops to 1 ounce of gel.

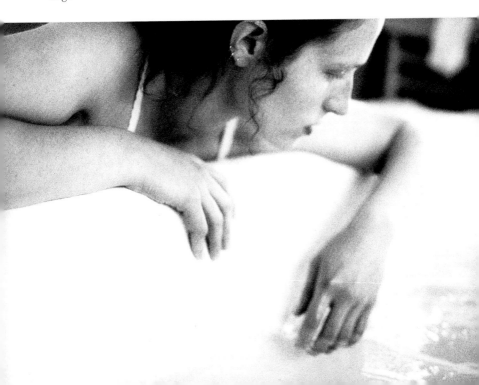

SUMMER BREEZES SOAK

Wrap the first four ingredients in a muslin bag and hang it from the faucet as your tub fills with water. Allow it to steep for five minutes. Then add the five oils to the bath, agitate the water, and submerge yourself!

1/4 cup organic rolled oats	1 tablespoon violet leaves	2 drops neroli
1 tablespoon orange blossoms	1 tablespoon lemon verbena leaves	1 drop geranium
	5 drops lemon	1 drop jasmine samboc
	3 drops red mandarin	

SUMMONING A CITRON AND VIOLET WOODLAND

Add the oils to 4 ounces of foaming bath or shower gel, preferably of a violet blue color to echo the violet fragrance. Shake extremely well, add a dollop to a natural sponge, and suds up.

7 drops sandalwood	2 drops mandarin	1 drop spikenard
5 drops pink grapefruit	petitgrain	1 drop basil
4 drops lime	2 drops ginger grass	1 drop violet leaf
3 drops rosemary	2 drops angelica root	
2 drops geranium	1 drop grand fir	

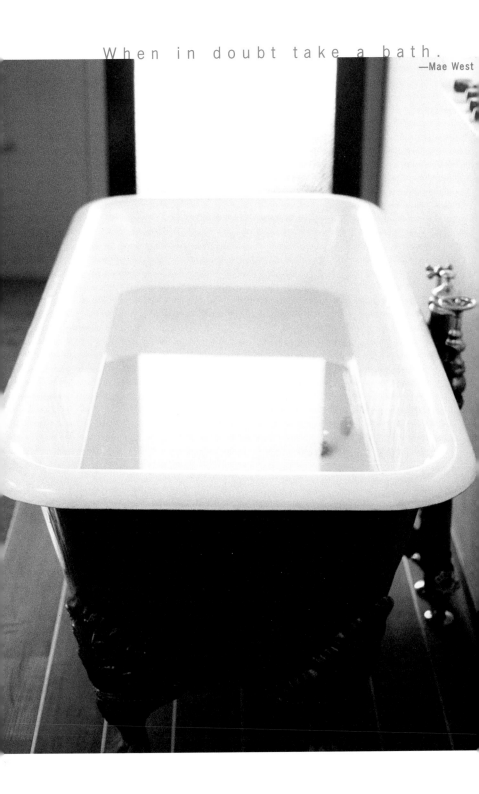

When in doubt take a bath.
—Mae West

MASSAGE

Massage is one of the most nurturing of alternative health and spa delights, as well as one of the most pleasurable and sensual shared experiences. Not only is the loving touch of massage therapeutic, but including an essential oil in the massage base can help rejuvenate the body by alleviating pain and muscle fatigue while lifting the spirits. When creating an aromatic massage lotion or oil, use a carrier base such as a cold-pressed, preferably organic seed, nut, or vegetal oil or an unscented unguent or cream to dispense the essential oils. Allow the carrier to come to room temperature, then add 10 to 15 drops of combined oils per ounce of the base. This dilution is at 1 to 2 percent. For pregnant women, infants, and the frail, use 5 drops per ounce. Before you apply the lotion or oil, remember to do a skin patch test on the person who will be receiving the massage.

---

dilution ratio table

At 2% to 5% depending on the strength you desire,
1 to 5 drops each to every 100 drops Base Oil

1 teaspoon = 5 milliliters

1 ounce = 30 milliliters

5 milliliters = 100 to 150 drops*

30 milliliters (1 ounce) = 600 to 900 drops*

Into 1 ounce or 30 millilite

1% = 6 to 9 drops

2% = 12 to 18 drops

3% = 18 to 27 drops

* depending on viscosity

MIDNIGHT SUN MASSAGE OIL

Blend the following essences into 2 ounces of pure, preferably organic vegetal oils such as hazelnut, sesame, and sweet almond, combined in equal portions.

10 drops red mandarin	2 drops ginger	1 drop cinnamon
5 drops vanilla CO_2	1 drop black pepper	
4 drops champaca	1 drop cardamom	

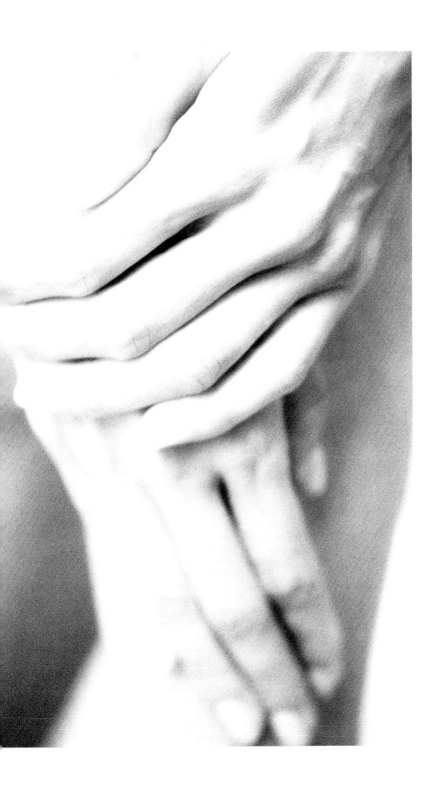

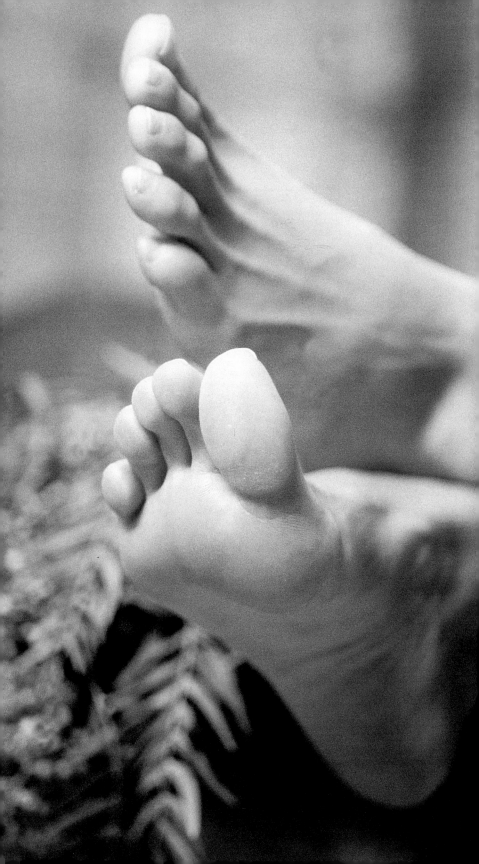

ARIEL'S REVIVE BODY SPRITZ

Add the grated organic orange peel to the vodka or grain alcohol and allow the mixture to steep in an airtight, diffused-glass receptacle in a cool cupboard for one week. Strain the mixture through fine, unbleached muslin or a coffee filter into another amber receptacle and add the oils. Blend in the rose hydrosol and distilled water and steep for two days. Strain into the original amber receptacle for storage. When you're ready to use, pour some of the mixture into an amber atomizer, shake well, and spritz sparingly.

1 ounce distilled water	1 tablespoon finely	5 drops lime
4 ounces rose hydrosol	grated organic	5 drops bergamot
1/2 ounce good vodka	orange peel	3 drops linden blossom
or grain alcohol	5 drops red mandarin	2 drops jasmine

foot massage

OWNING YOUR FEET

6 drops lavender

3 drops marjoram

2 drops rose attar

1 drop violet leaf

1 drop spearmint

1 drop thyme

The Greek physician Hippocrates believed that the path to optimal health begins with a daily aromatic bath and scented massage. To this, I would add a weekly aromatherapeutic foot massage and pampering. In a deep-welled aromatic burner, warm 1 to 2 tablespoons of an unscented base oil, and add 4 to 6 drops of an essential oil or synergy. Slowly work the oil into your feet, concentrating on the soles. Try lavender to create a sense of equilibrium and relaxation, chamomile to ease swollen feet, peppermint to rejuvenate and balance a tired disposition, rosemary for stiffness or pain, or black pepper to enhance circulation.

facial massage

BLOSSOMED EXOTICA

5 drops neroli

3 drops red mandarin

2 drops rose attar

2 drops linden blossom

2 drops sandalwood

1 drop jasmine samboc

1 drop frankincense

A facial massage can soothe problem skin, relieve a headache, and ease nasal problems such as sinusitis. Some experts believe it can even prevent premature aging of the skin. To make a facial oil, add 3 to 5 drops of a synergy to $\frac{1}{3}$ ounce unscented base oil or lotion. Shake to combine. For dry skin, try sandalwood or chamomile; for normal skin, try lavender or geranium; for oily skin, try lemon or clary sage.

A BEE'S WHISPER TONER OR AFTERSHAVE

Combine the vodka, honey, and essential oils in a small, sterile diffused-glass bottle. Let the combination mature for seven to 12 days, gently shaking often. Then pour into a 4-ounce integrated-color glass atomizer filled with 3 ounces of distilled water and add the rosemary hydrosol. Add more distilled water if needed until the container is full.

3 ounces distilled water	3 drops lime petitgrain	2 tablespoons rosemary
2 tablespoons vodka	3 drops yuzu	hydrosol
1/4 teaspoon honey	2 drops cardamom	
4 drops neroli	1 drop vetiver	

HOUSEHOLD applications

Essential oils can work their magic throughout the home, scenting your days and sweetening your chores. Their uses extend as far as your imagination, but here are a few suggestions to start you off. Keep an atomizer filled with water and a synergy of essences such as lavender, lemon, and tea tree, and use it to wipe down counters, tubs, and sinks. Place 1 to 3 drops of an oil such as lavender onto the side of your toilet paper roll. Add 1 to 3 drops of an oil such as eucalyptus, fir, or grapefruit to the rinse cycle of your washing machine. Place cotton balls scented with a drop of rose attar or sweet orange in your lingerie drawer, jasmine or sandalwood in your pillowcase at night, vetiver or violet leaf between the pages of your books, and cardamom or lemon in stale cupboards. Place cotton balls scented with peppermint in corners, under porch steps, and on windowsills to ward off pests and insects.

FOREST AND HONEY ROOM SPRAY

In a small porcelain bowl, blend 1 teaspoon of the vodka with the oakmoss, vetiver, and violet leaf, and stir with an untreated wooden toothpick. Add the other essences and stir again. Pour the distilled water and the rest of the vodka into an integrated-color glass atomizer and add the contents of the bowl. Shake well and spritz sparingly.

5 1/2 ounces distilled water	5 drops champaca	3 drops altas cedarwood
1/2 ounce vodka or grain alcohol	3 drops black spruce	3 drops vetiver
	3 drops grand fir	2 drops violet leaf
	3 drops silver fir	1 drop oakmoss

LEMONED AND RUBIED GLEN PLANT SPRAY

Each year at the beginning of spring and the end of summer I create this rejuvenating spray for my houseplants. Fill half a 7.5-milliliter (1/2 ounce) amber vial with citrus oils (I like to include lemon and yellow mandarin in the spring and red mandarin and pink grapefruit in the fall), then add a blending of conifer oils (my favorites include grand fir, silver fir, a touch of sitka spruce, rocky mountain juniper in spring) until the synergy is pleasing to your nose. Add 8 to 10 drops to a 2-ounce spray bottle filled with distilled water and 2 or 3 drops of liquid soap, spray this mixture onto the leaves of all your plants, and dry with a soft cotton cloth. You will be amazed at how clean and aromatic your environment will become. Your body will feel revived and energized, the cobwebs will clear from your mind, and your spirit will be replenished.

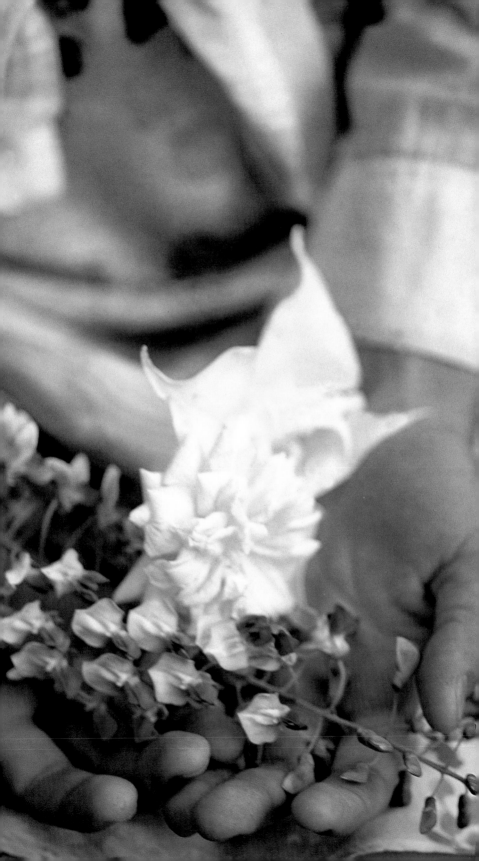

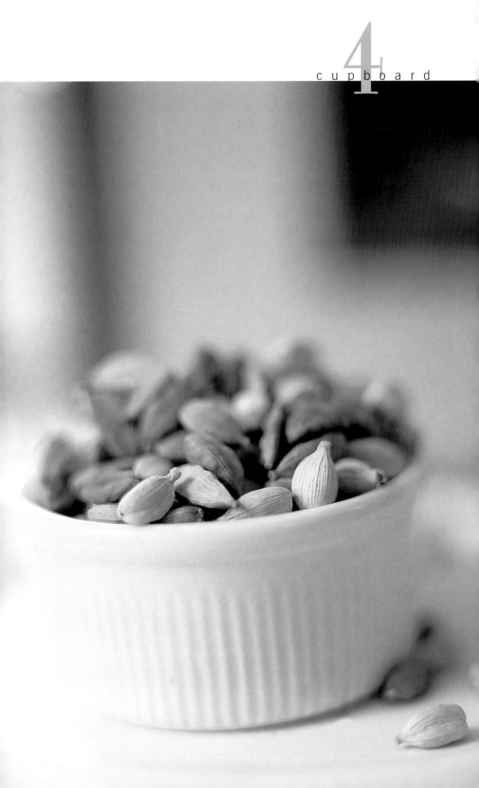

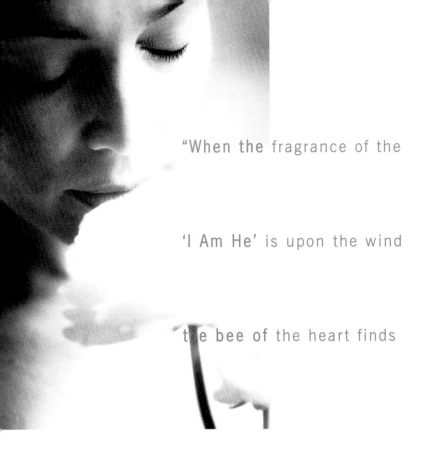

"When the fragrance of the

'I Am He' is upon the wind

the bee of the heart finds

the flower of its choice

and nestles there,

caring for no other thing."
—Kabir

The Egyptians believed that the nose was the portal to the soul. The power of aromatherapy lies in the fact that essential oils not only have chemical structures that allow them to heal our bodies, they possess unrivaled aromas with the ability to alter our emotions and move our spirit. All too often in modern-day medicine, physicians treat physical symptoms without recognizing the correlation between the body, mind, and soul. But those of us who are students of the natural healing arts know that healing begins with the health and strength of one's mind and the refinement and peace of one's soul.

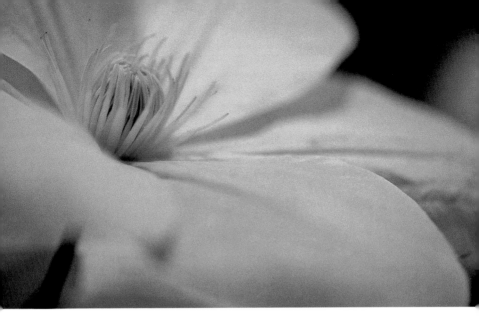

In this chapter, I present you with the beginnings of an aromatic cupboard, consisting of nine Basic Oils and ten Sensuous Oils. Although
all of these essences are graced with aromatic distinction, the basic
oils have been chosen because they form a beginner's apothecary,
while the sensuous oils have been chosen for their aromatic splendor.
This is not to say, however, that the sensuous oils are merely pleasing
to the nose. Although many of the sensuous oils are absolutes, which
are rarely used by aromatherapists, the essential oils among them—
cardamom, clary sage, black pepper, rosemary, sandalwood, and
vetiver—afford invaluable therapeutic benefits, and the reader is
encouraged to explore the wide range of their applications further.

As you build your cupboard, you will embark on a wonderful
aromatic adventure. As I try to convey to my clients and students,
beyond the body there lies the spirit, beyond the mind there lies the
emotions, beyond the practical there lies the aesthetic, and beyond
the fundamental there lies the sensual.

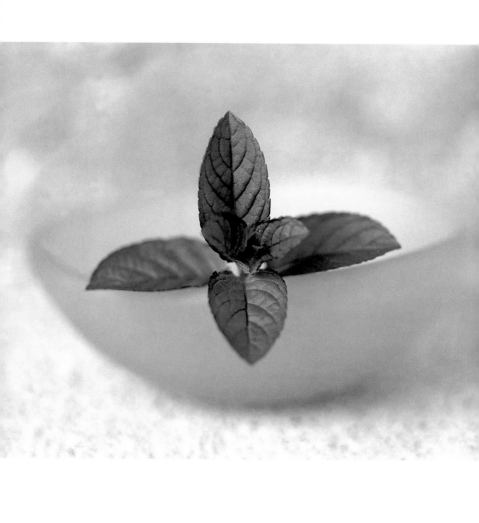

THE BASIC OILS

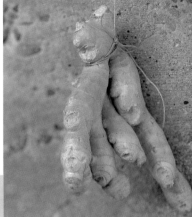

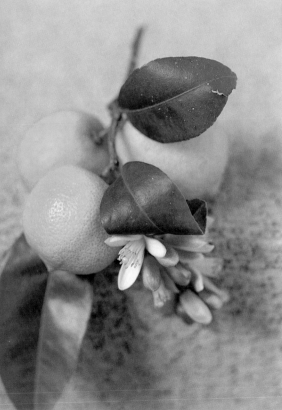

Roman Chamomile

Eucalyptus

Geranium

Ginger

Lavender

Lemon

Mandarin Orange

Peppermint

Tea Tree

roman
·chamomile

(Chamaemelum nobile/Anthemis nobilis)

Traditionally in England, chamomile was trodden into the floor to delicately scent the home. Perhaps it was this simple act rising out of humble households that afforded chamomile its reputation as the herb of modesty and humility.

Roman chamomile is native to southern and western Europe and is naturalized in North America. The oil is extracted by steam distillation of the flower heads. True Roman chamomile—not to be confused with Moroccan or German chamomile—can be recognized by its pale blue tint. Its scent is fruity, reminiscent of a ripe apple, pungently herbal, and spicy. In fact, it takes its name from the root of the Greek word *khamaimelon*, and more recently, from the Spanish word *manzanilla*, both of which refer to "little apple."

Chamomile supports the blood and the nervous, musculoskeletal, endocrine (hormonally), digestive, and eliminatory systems. It is one of the few essential oils that reduces the effects of allergies. It is used for maladies from asthma to arthritis, burns to fever. It relieves the symptoms of menopause and treats numerous skin disorders.

Emotionally, chamomile fosters calmness and ease. It is an antidote to stress, insomnia, anger, irrationality, impulsiveness, oversensitivity, and short-temperedness. Because it is nontoxic and nonirritating, it is a perfect oil to use with children. It will calm tantrums and foster a quiet night's sleep.

Avoid using chamomile in the first trimester of pregnancy. It has been reported that long-term use should be avoided with estrogen-dependent cancers. And always use it in a low dilution, such as 1 percent. A maximum of 3 to 5 drops is recommended in 1 to 2 teaspoons of a base product or in a bath.

eucalyptus

(Eucalyptus globulus)

The eucalyptus is one of the world's tallest trees. Medicinally, it was first employed by the aboriginal peoples of Australia, primarily to treat wounds. Its name derives from the Greek word *eucalyptos*, which means "well-covered," referring to the caplike membrane that covers the tree's tiny white flowers when they are in full bloom.

There are more than 700 species of eucalyptus, 500 of which produce an essential oil. Native to Tasmania, Australia, and China, eucalyptus is now also cultivated in Spain, Portugal, and California. Extraction is by steam distillation from fresh or partially dried leaves and young twigs. The scent of eucalyptus is piercing and camphoraceous, with an undertone of sweet wood. Freshly extracted oil is usually colorless, but the oil may yellow with age.

Eucalyptus supports respiration—the renewal of oxygen to the lungs. It relieves asthma, bronchitis, and sinus and throat infection, and in general strengthens our immune system. Because it has muscular and circulatory affinity, it also treats rheumatism and can relieve skin irritations such as boils, blisters, blemishes, cold sores, and insect bites. Eucalyptus helps restore alertness and reduces mood swings. It increases optimism and openness, and will cool a hot temper.

Always dilute eucalyptus when using it on the skin. Avoid it altogether if you have a history of epilepsy or hypertension, and don't employ it in conjunction with homeopathic remedies. Eucalyptus has been reported to be toxic when ingested. A maximum of 1 to 3 drops is recommended in 1 to 2 teaspoons of a base product or in a bath.

geranium

Arab legend tells how Mohammed hung his freshly washed shirt out to dry on a mallow plant. Being of the humblest of origins, the mallow blushed profusely in shades of crimson and pink and thus was transformed into geranium.

Geranium is native to southern and western Europe and is naturalized in North America. It represents a family of 500 species.

When buying an oil, look for the *Pelargonium* genus. The oil's scent is earthy, sweet, and green with interlacing minty and roselike tones. It is extracted by steam distillation from the leaves, stalks, and flowers—the whole plant is aromatic. The oil's color is pale olive green.

Geranium was highly valued by Native Americans to treat conditions ranging from toothache to cholera. Today it is considered an antidiabetic oil and a lymphatic stimulant. It is used to relieve PMS and symptoms of menopause; and is a vital skin care component in treating disorders such as chicken pox, measles, dermatitis, and eczema; even ulcers and tumors. It can also be a superb insect repellent.

Geranium is sometimes nicknamed the "mediator oil." It is thought to harmonize and balance the emotions and help draw an even ground between disputing parties. It is an especially adaptive oil, with the ability to address a wide variety of emotional and physical needs. It can strengthen feelings of security, receptivity, and intimacy, and neutralize fear and depression.

Avoid geranium if you are recently pregnant. It has been reported that long-term use should be avoided with estrogen-dependent cancer. You may also want to avoid it at bedtime; in some people it causes insomnia and restlessness. A maximum of 3 to 4 drops is recommended in 1 to 2 teaspoons of a base product or in a bath.

ginger.

According to the Koran, ginger was served at the meals in paradise, and is now nicknamed the Paradise Flower. When the Red Sea trade routes opened, the Arabs were among the first to make ginger available to the Greeks and Romans, who considered the spice as valuable as gold. The Roman philosopher Avicenna perfected its distillation and recommended its use, dispensed in a honeyed syrup, to treat impotence. In the 12th century, the healer St. Hildegard von Bingen touted its efficacy as an aphrodisiac.

Today India and Jamaica produce some of the best ginger. The essence is extracted by steam distillation from the unpeeled, dried, ground rhizome, after the flower stem has dried off. The aroma is tenacious and warm, slightly citrus, green, and spicy. Its color is pale yellow or green and is also available in CO_2 form.

Ginger is still used as an aphrodisiac today. It is a metabolic booster; it raises the body temperature, increases circulation, and relieves muscle strain. In fact, *Doctrine of Signatures*, which is a manual that correlates a plant with the organ of the body it supports, connects ginger with the entire digestive system. It is a well-known antidote for loss of appetite and nausea and is often used to treat jet lag and travel sickness. It is also used to treat colds, respiratory infection, and influenza. It is said to be effective in the treatment of liver congestion and heart disease. Ginger also curbs exhaustion and increases self-confidence and initiative.

Ginger can irritate the skin and can be slightly phototoxic. Be cautious with its topical use, especially on inflamed skin or near the face. Avoid it altogether if you have bleeding ulcers, gallstones, or a high fever. A maximum of 1 to 3 drops is recommended in 1 to 2 teaspoons of a base product or in a bath.

·lavender

Lavender is a derivative of the Latin word *lavare*, which means "to wash." It was a ritual bathing herb in Roman times, and in the 12th century St. Hildegard von Bingen became widely known for her healing lavender water. In ancient Greece, lavender was dedicated to Hecate and believed to ward off the evil eye. In North Africa, it was purported to avert wild cats and even a spouse's mistreatment.

Today lavender is cultivated all over the world, especially in England, France, Bulgaria, and the United States. Lavender oil is extracted by steam distillation from the fresh flowering tops of the plant. Its scent is camphoraceously sweet and herbaceously floral with rich balsamic wood undertones. The oil's color is clear pale yellow. *Lavendula officinalis* (*angustifolia*) is the favorite of aromatherapists because of its aromatic warmth and richness and its versatility.

Lavender is considered an anti-allergic and an antibiotic oil. It can help lower blood pressure, balance the blood sugar, and assuredly ease minor aches and pains. It inhibits the growth of bacteria on the skin while stimulating the growth of healthy cells, making it highly beneficial for wound care. It is supportive to all skin types and applicable to afflictions such as blisters, bites, and burns. It affects the emotions by soothing irritability and apprehension. It calms the spirit, balances one's disposition, and inspires self-expression. Lavender is one of the most effective oils when used for children's bumps and scrapes, even easing their fears of the dark.

Lavender should not be used in preparations containing iron or iodine. Avoid it in the first trimester of pregnancy and if you have low blood pressure. A maximum of 3 to 6 drops is recommended in 1 to 2 teaspoons of a base product or in a bath. Lavender is susceptible to hydrolysis and oxidation, which diminish its shelf life, so it should be stored carefully.

lemon·

I think of lemon essence as bottled sunshine. A single tree may produce up to 2,000 lemons, but since it takes as many as 1,500 lemons to produce a single pound of essential oil, lemon is almost as precious as liquid gold.

There are close to 50 varieties of lemon grown throughout the world, and some of the highest quality oil originates in Sicily. Lemon oil is cold expressed from the outer part of the fresh peel. Its color is a pale yellow-green that turns brown with age. Its scent is reminiscent of the peel—bright, sharp, crisp, and with the characteristic tang of citrus.

In ancient Europe, lemons were considered a cure-all for infectious diseases. The full range of the fruit's medicinal uses was established by the pharmacist Nicholas Lemery in the early 17th century. By the 20th century, the components of lemon oil in vapor form when inhaled were shown to be effective in the treatment of numerous viral and bacterial infections. Still today, lemon is commonly used to stimulate the immune system, as it activates both red and white blood cell formation. It can help lower blood pressure, aid digestion, support weight management, reduce varicose veins and cellulite, and even detoxify vital eliminatory organs.

Lemon is an adatagenic oil, and as such, balances the physical, emotional, mental, and spiritual planes. It alleviates lethargy, curtails resentment and bitterness, and fosters concentration and self-expression.

When using lemon on the skin, avoid overexposure to the sun, as the oil may be phototoxic. Avoid the oil altogether if you have sensitive skin or are allergic to citrus fruits. A maximum of 3 to 6 drops is recommended in 1 to 2 teaspoons of a base product or in a bath. Lemon will keep for only six to eight months, so renew your supply often.

·mandarin orange

(Citrus reticulata var. mandarin, Citrus madurensis, Citrus nobilis)

Varieties of *Citrus reticulata* found in the United States are oftentimes incorrectly referred to as tangerine. The oil of tangerine is a pale melon-yellow, whereas mandarin is a deep shade of golden amber with a distinctive hue of blue luminescence. While both oils are deliciously sweet and tangy, the scent of tangerine has a crisp airy freshness that mandarin replaces with an opulent warm depth and floral undertones. Some of the loveliest mandarin essential oil is sourced from the Mediterranean.

Mandarin oil has been extensively studied for appropriate application to a vast spectrum of distresses to the digestive and excretory systems. In times of stress, when the liver is under duress, it has been shown to support better assimilation of fats, which can otherwise often lead to tension headaches and insomnia.

Mandarin is a beautiful oil for spa; an immune and lymphatic stimulant, it also supports tissue regeneration and detoxification, reduces scarring and stretch marks, and is used to nurture dry and aging skin.

It may have gained its resolute reputation of being an oil of calm reserve because of the fruit's bromine-rich composition, which is a natural sedative. Joyful and positive in its expression, it can quickly overcome moodiness and irritation. It is a gentle oil for children, and offers women emotional and physical support throughout pregnancy. It is said that you can easily "give yourself a hug" through a deep inhalation of mandarin essence.

When using mandarin on the skin, avoid overexposure to the sun, since the oil can be phototoxic. Avoid the oil altogether if you are allergic to citrus fruits. A maximum of 3 to 5 drops is recommended in 1 to 2 teaspoons of a base product or in a bath. On the shelf, mandarin will keep for only six to eight months, so renew your supply often.

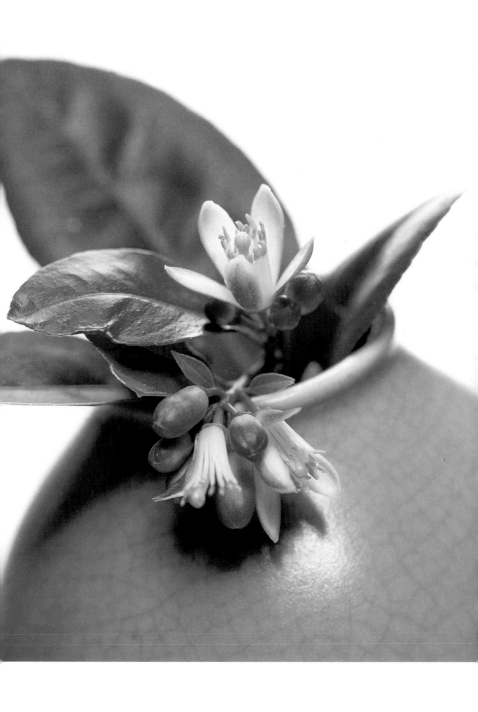

·peppermint

(Mentha piperita)

In Greek mythology, when the god Pluto fell in love with the beautiful nymph Mentha, his jealous wife Persephone turned her into a plant to be trod upon. But to ease his broken heart, Pluto transformed her into the aromatic healing herb mint, one of today's most familiar essences. We find mint everywhere: in toothpaste, breath freshener, candy, gum, and beverages.

Peppermint is native to Europe, Brazil, and the United States. Its oil is extracted by steam distillation from the flowering herb. Its aroma is a piercing camphoraceous grassy mint on a balsamic base, and its color is pale yellow-green.

The use of peppermint is recorded in the most ancient of surviving medical texts, the Ebers papyrus. The cooling and warming effects of peppermint's menthol make it a wonderful overall tonic, helpful for everything from muscle strain to stomachaches to dizziness to jet lag; it even relieves the itch of chicken pox. It makes an ideal treatment for the aches and pains of illness and of overactivity. Peppermint's invigorating scent is a quick pick-me-up. It refreshes the spirit, aids the memory, and spurs the thought process.

Peppermint may slow the milk production of nursing mothers, so avoid it during lactation. Also avoid it when using homeopathic medications and if you have epilepsy or heart disease. It has been known to cause allergic reactions in the throat and mouth. In some cases it may aggravate chills with fever, and it may have an adverse affect on young children. A maximum of 1 to 3 drops is recommended in 1 to 2 teaspoons of a base product or in a bath.

tea tree

Tea tree is the general term for members of the Melaleuca family. Its name derives from its use as an herbal tea. Our present-day incorporation of Melaleuca oils in therapy is based on a long history of use by the aboriginal peoples of Australia. Research has found tea tree to be unique in its immune-stimulant properties, which are effective against our three primary infectious organisms—bacterial, fungal, and viral. Even so, it was not until 1933 that the *British Medical Journal* gave tea tree the recognition it so justly deserves. The essential oil is steam- or water-distilled from the leaves and twigs of the tree. Its aroma is petrol sharp, camphoraceous, waxen, and medicinal. Its color is pale yellow-green or water-white.

While other potent antiseptic oils can be irritating or even damaging to the skin, pure tea tree is not. It is good for treating bug bites and can be used to fight ticks, leeches, lice, and fungus. In fact, it is perfect for abrasions and infections of all kinds. It will also aid with respiratory complaints, asthma, and catarrh, and in general acts as a support to the immune system. Tea tree's effect on the mind is stimulating and uplifting. It helps clear the head, prevents exhaustion, proves beneficial in times of shock, and curbs perfectionism.

Overuse of tea tree can be toxic to animals, and in some people it may irritate the skin. Perform a patch test before incorporating it in topical applications. A maximum of 1 to 4 drops is recommended in 1 to 2 teaspoons of a base product or in a bath.

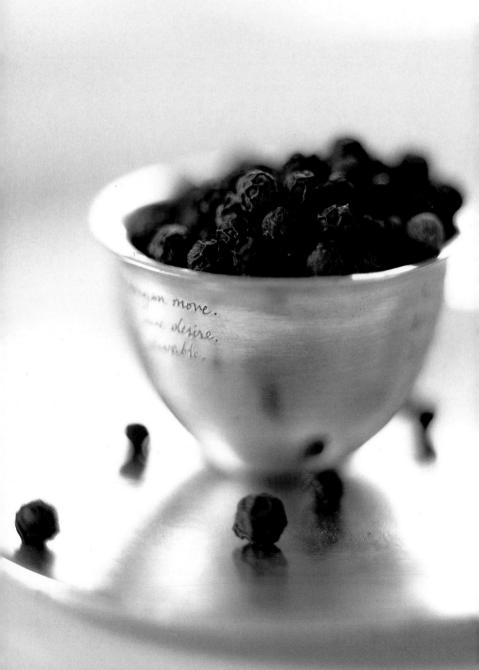

THE SENSUOUS OILS

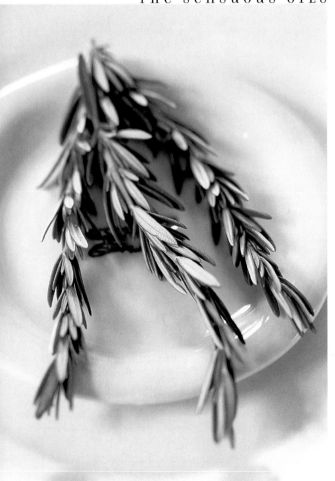

Cardamom

Clary Sage

Jasmine

Linden Blossom

Black Pepper

Rosemary

Sandalwood

Vanilla

Vetiver

Violet Leaf

cardamom

A quick sniff of cardamom is not enough to enjoy its full effect; one must inhale it deeply and fully. This is the only way to experience the unparalleled complexity of cardamom's lilting, fragrant camphoric spices intertwined with its sweet pungent ribbons of dry wood and silken honey balsam in the same moment.

Exotic cousin to the ginger plant, cardamom is native to, and principally cultivated in, the humid, woody hillsides and forests of southwest India, Sri Lanka, Southeast Asia, and Guatemala. After Hippocrates documented its medicinal value, cardamom became an "essential" spice sold by Viking and Portuguese traders. Subsequently, it was found to be an honored element in recipes for liqueurs and perfumes.

Many cooks revere black pepper as the "king" of spices, and cardamom is rightfully acknowledged to be the "queen." Cleopatra herself lavishly scented her chambers with its sweet aphrodisiac scent. It was a lucky choice for her seduction of Mark Antony, for cardamom inspires a sense of courage as well as sensual enthusiasm.

We could all benefit from the modern-day Bedouin practice of lacing hot milk and coffee with this time-honored spice. Vitally supportive to the digestive system, cardamom has the reputation of countering the digestive effects of caffeine and of our dairy-laden Western diet. Cardamom is most beneficial for renewing a sense of one's center and connectedness to the earth. It spurs physical activity while adding fuel to our passions.

Cardamom can be phototoxic, and it should be avoided in the first trimester of pregnancy. A maximum of 1 to 2 drops is recommended in 2 to 4 teaspoons of a base product or in a bath.

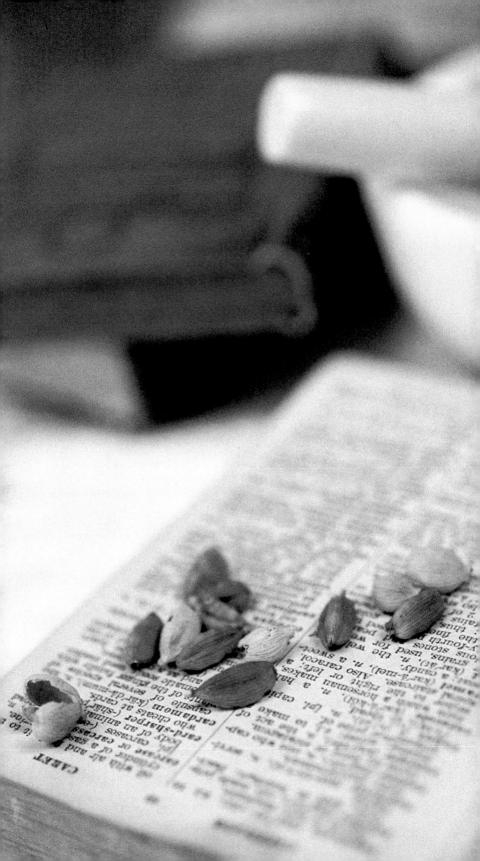

·clary sage

(Salvia sclarea)

I remember well the first time I sat near a patch of these aggressive yet graceful bushlike plants. Dotted with blossoms in spring pastels, they appeared to have been splashed gingerly yet deliberately by a painter's brush. Even though I was in an urban setting, the air smelled as if there were a pasture nearby.

In the heat of the day, clary sage emits a scent very much like its bottled essence. A lilting herbal sweetness meets your nostrils carrying the slight startle of pungent camphor combined with the warmth of hay, hinting at mustiness that has been rolled into a nutty layering.

Clary sage originated in the warm Mediterranean. Now it is cultivated throughout Europe, the United States, and Canada. The Pacific Northwest in particular produces some excellent clary sage oil, which is steamed distilled from the flowering herb.

The charm of clary sage is that it does not remove us from the present moment. We remain steadfastly earthbound while our senses are recharged and reawakened. Clary sage brushes away elusive cobwebs and allows for clear thoughts and decisiveness. It stills our minds and allows us to receive messages and directions that are otherwise shrouded by worry and stress. By dispelling our anxieties and allowing us to access our wisdom, clary sage gives us the opportunity to relish the moment. Drawing us to a center of calm, it opens a doorway to the endless possibility of being in touch with ourselves, as well as with each other.

Clary sage is considered a narcotic and should be used with care. Avoid it during the first trimester of pregnancy. Also, it may cause headache and should be avoided if you have estrogen-related health problems. A maximum of 2 to 5 drops is recommended in 1 to 2 teaspoons of a base product or in a bath.

jasmine

Indian folklore tells of a beautiful princess who fell hopelessly in love with the God of the Sun. Tormented when he rejected her, she took her own life, and the ground upon which her ashes were scattered sprouted a glorious jasmine bush. Honoring her demise, the jasmine's miniature starlike blossoms would forever reject the warm rays of the sun to choose instead the cool of the night, under the light of the moon, to emit their heavenly essence.

The jasmine flower is imbued with an odor tapestry so rich that it could easily be the envy of the floral kingdom. Rising up indolic-sharp, its aroma spirals down into a luscious honey-tea floral and ends in a scent of green ambrosia. *Jasminum grandiflorum* has a heady sugared warmth, *Jasminum sambac* a green fruitiness.

Jasmine's flowers begin to open at dusk and are harvested near sunrise, before any damage can occur as the result of the morning dew. It takes nearly 40 pounds of precious petals to obtain a single ounce of jasmine essence, which is commonly available as a concrete and an absolute. Along with rose, jasmine is one of the most expensive, yet one of the most essential, flowers of perfumery.

Jasmine promotes a state of relaxation that can relieve physical discomfort that is the result of a psychological or emotional imbalance. It elevates us to a higher state of consciousness that allows us to accept life's experiences, encouraging self-confidence and unleashing stagnating energy. It is revered as the oil of hope and optimistic renewal, and it can diminish the inhibitions that often lead us to hold in reserve our longing to share physically, barring no restraints, with another.

Claims have been made that jasmine is one of the most common allergens in perfumery and may affect dermatologically sensitive individuals. A maximum of 1 to 2 drops is recommended in 1 to 2 teaspoons of a base product or in a bath.

linden blossom

If ever the smell of summer was captured in an essence, it is that of the delicate linden blossom. Clusters of linden blooms emanate a symphony of honeyed vanilla floral, cascading over voluptuous undertones of sweet, somewhat green cantaloupe melon teased with a hint of tang reminiscent of lime. I defy anyone to abide in crossness or worry upon inhaling linden's sweetly balanced fruited and floral tranquillity.

In Greek mythology, the mighty god Zeus helped Philemon and Baucis preserve their love by transforming one into an oak and the other into a linden tree. Ever since, the linden has remained a symbol of fidelity and undying love. Historically, linden, which is not an essential oil, but a concrete or absolute, has been applied therapeutically for matters of the heart. It is believed to increase our connection with others and soften communication. It helps cure lovesickness, depression, nervousness, insomnia, and vertigo. Linden's emollient qualities make it the perfect addition to body creams, lotions, and soaps.

When I am searching to perfect a synergy of oils, it is regularly the flower oils, such as linden, to which I turn. A beautiful complement to a blend, linden also remains unshakably complete in itself. Its exotic strength and innocent sensuality allows the mind to become calm and still and gives the sense of wings sprouting from the soul, affording our expressions of love a childlike playfulness and gaiety.

Linden may cause skin irritation, especially if used undiluted without a carrier. A maximum of 1 to 2 drops is recommended in 1 to 2 teaspoons of a base product or in a bath.

black pepper

(Piper nigrum)

Black pepper has a scent with the ability to move mountains. Its top notes of green emanate from a warm, spiced heart that evolves into a lemon balsam and exits on a note of piquant dry wood shavings. Pepper is a true catalyst to initiate action. A mere whiff affords a sense of comfort while encouraging strength, fearlessness, and increased vigor and stamina.

A pepper plant must be established for four years before it will form berries ripe for harvest. A true exotic, pepper grows in India, Indochina, Indonesia, Madagascar, the Comoro Islands, and Thailand, and tons of the precious fruit are exported yearly to all parts of the world. The berries of the plant are dried, crushed, and steam distilled to create the essential oil. But steam destroys much of the tenacious piquantness of spice berries and this essential oil deteriorates quickly, affording a short shelf life unless stored well. It is the robust unripe black pepper berries that are most often distilled into oil, but the subtle green pepper oil has its own magical effervescence.

There is rarely a blend that cannot be enhanced, even made somewhat divine, by the interweaving of black pepper. Its aromatic spiciness can arouse a sense of curiosity and rekindle a flame of passion that has flickered to an ebb. It is a true athlete's companion, with warming and stimulating properties that combat pain, inflammation, stiffness, and overall fatigue. This was the oil that ancient Romans used to send warriors into battle, as well as into the boudoir.

Use black pepper in moderation; it has been reported that excessive use may cause kidney troubles. It can also be irritating to sensitive skin. A maximum of 1 to 3 drops is recommended in 1 to 2 teaspoons of a base product or in a bath.

·rosemary

(Rosmarinus officinalis)

If ever there was an essence that enhanced one's sense of ego, strength, and the ability to "go the distance," it is rosemary. A mere whiff sets the mind, body, and spirit in order and provides the gratifying sense that all is right with the world. Piercing, strong, hearty, warm, pungent, and rich all in the same breath, rosemary is distinctively laden with notes of mint and balsamic wood along with incensed honey, giving it the textured characteristics of a sun-drenched woodland.

Linked with the ancient divinity of Apollo, rosemary seems to elicit, as the vision of Apollo must have, a sense of confidence. Its fiery herbaceous notes conjure a feeling of purpose, potential, and personal destiny. As an herb of the sun, rosemary happily resides in the warm climes of the Mediterranean, but this evergreen herb has a hardiness that makes it fairly adaptable throughout the world.

Rosemary is not an herb reserved for youth; it also offers mature users a sense of grace and rejuvenation. It is used to reduce signs of aging such as gray hair, hair loss, and wrinkles. It was one of the essential ingredients in the famous Hungary water that was concocted for Queen Isabella, who at the age of 70 married the much younger king of Poland.

An Old World ritual was to tuck sprigs of rosemary into newlyweds' shoes to symbolize their infinite fidelity to each other. Thus, rosemary has borne the reputation of an herb of constancy, trust, and loyalty.

Use rosemary moderately. Do not use it for steam inhalation if you are asthmatic. Avoid it altogether if you are pregnant or breast-feeding, of if you have hypertension, epilepsy, or a distressed liver. It is best applied diluted and should not be used with small children. A maximum of 2 to 4 drops is recommended in 1 to 2 teaspoons of a base product or in a bath.

sandalwood·

(Santalam album)

An oil highly valued in ancient times for religious purposes, sandalwood was used in embalming, because it was thought that its scent escorted the departed spirit to its new life. Today, sandalwood paste is still rubbed between the eyebrows to distinguish followers of the Hindu faith. Because this spot is a central nerve relay point, this denotation of religious choice also adeptly gives its wearer the demeanor of serenity and strength throughout the day, fostering temperance, patience, and love.

The distillation of sandalwood remains an important livelihood in India and is one of that country's most treasured products. The high demand for sandalwood oil has put restraints on its cultivation, which is now controlled by the government. It takes nearly 25 pounds of the precious heartwood to produce a pound of essential oil. Therefore, it should be sourced carefully and used in small quantities and with great reverence.

Like a sea of amber honey, sandalwood's notes tumble and roll, encircling us in sensual warmth and joy. Heavily laden with velvety notes of wood and tinged with hints of exotic fruit, it has no discernible top note, but begins at a pungent and rich middle and flows evenly into shavings of sweetly powdered wood.

In a synergy, sandalwood plays the role of custodian, instilling a smooth, even balance to the blend. It is used for meditation and is a primary ingredient in the erotic recipes of the *Kama Sutra*. Sandalwood can connect us to the divinity that lies deep within ourselves. By screening out external strife, it creates a sense of interconnectedness and allows us to creatively embrace and selflessly savor the love that we seek to experience in our daily lives.

Sandalwood is generally nontoxic and nonirritating, but long-term use may adversely affect the liver. A maximum of 2 to 4 drops is recommended in 1 to 2 teaspoons of a base product or in a bath.

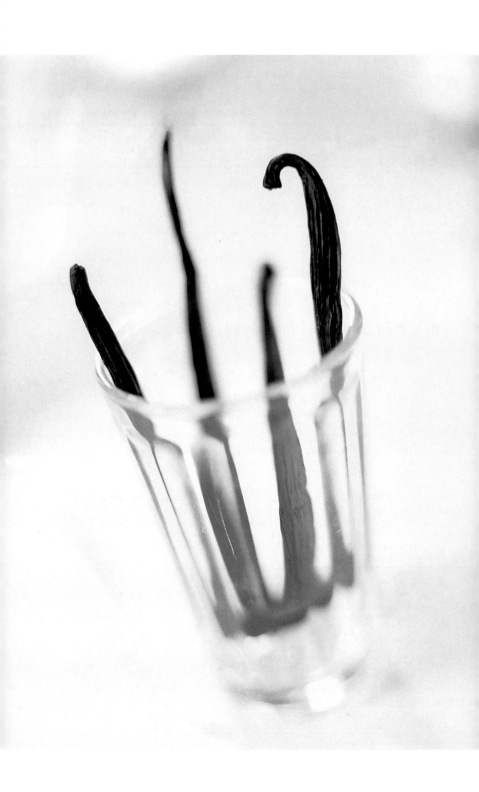

Who can turn away from the unrivaled scent of vanilla? Who can remain unmoved by such a confectionery aroma with the ability to conjure a sense of space similar to the calm at the eye of the storm. Once touted as a mental stimulant, yet contrarily rumored to be a narcotic, vanilla conjures a feeling of free-spirited opulence while at the same time creating the comfort of immeasurable security.

In the wild, the climbing vanilla vine attaches aerial rootings firmly to the trunks and limbs of neighboring trees and deliberately pulls itself skyward to bask in the rays of the warm sun. Although it produces fruit that can be cured to impeccable sweetness, its seafoam-yellow orchid blossoms are mysteriously without scent. Madagascar leads the cultivation and harvesting of vanilla beans by producing nearly a million pounds of the fragrant pods a year, but some of the highest quality vanilla beans come from Tahiti and Costa Rica.

A good vanilla essence will afford its audience a refrain of warmed caramels, root beer, browned sugar, sweet balsamic honey, and hickory smoke in one harmonious synergy. An aroma often linked with chocolate, vanilla creates a similar emotional response, offering refuge from irritation, frustration, anger, tension, and angst. Although Aztec men used vanilla to flavor their heated chocolate and drank it in copious amounts, they forbade their women to do the same, fearing its aftereffects too tantalizing and provocative! The theory that chocolate releases the same chemicals in the brain as sensual intimacy makes me wonder if the sugared balm notes of vanilla act as the precursor to such reactions.

Vanilla is nontoxic, yet it may be irritating to sensitive skin. A maximum of 1 to 2 drops is recommended in 1 to 2 teaspoons of a base product or in a bath.

·vetiver

Through the pressures of daily living, does your spirit seek to rise and soar? Then by all means grab a vial of the venerable oil of vetiver. Its essence, even in the smallest quantity, is laden with the heavily spiced, pungent mustiness of the earth. Vetiver often opens with a grassy top note, then unfurls to tantalize your nose with layer upon resinous layer of moist, wooded smokiness amidst the scent of steamy air that emanates from the floor of a hot tropical forest edged by marshland.

The resilient perennial grasses of vetiver can sustain the weather of tropical zones and are also adaptable to mountainous hillsides. Its meshing of rootlets, from which its oil is obtained, holds fast to soil that would otherwise be flushed away by torrential rains. The plant is used by indigenous populations for thatching and weaving, leaving only a couple of tons a year for essential oil production. It takes nearly 200 pounds of vetiver roots to produce one pound of the ambered aromatic oil, which should not be scorched in distillation.

Dubbed the "oil of tranquility," vetiver promotes not only a sense of serenity but also a feeling of substance, strength, and fortitude. It has the ability through its warm embrace to gather and reserve energy that is scattered or on the edge of depletion. It restores a feeling of capability and revives a sense of purpose. Sanskrit texts recommend vetiver for the chambers of newlyweds. Perhaps that is because it is the essence that eases our otherwise restless and detached natures and returns us to a keen self-awareness that allows us to attend with sensitivity and adeptness to our partners' needs.

Vetiver is generally nontoxic and nonirritating, but it may cause skin irritation in some individuals. It has been reported that excessive use may cause liver distress. A maximum of 1 to 2 drops is recommended in 1 to 2 teaspoons of a base product or in a bath.

violet leaf·

Many believe that it takes a trained nose to fully appreciate violet's delectable odor. Shakespeare called it "the perfume and suppliance of a minute." I disagree. Although the aroma of violet may be elusive, the moment you bury your nose in a tiny bundle of flowers, their scent will forever leave their impression, not only upon your mind, but upon your psyche. It is little wonder that ancient Athens, so steeped in virility and endurance, chose the bold little violet as its flower of distinction.

Violet leaf is the captured odor of rain-drenched moss and maple sugar, tumbled together with the peels of lemon and green birch bark, then allowed to dry in the half-shaded rays of midday sun. It is said that the best time to pick a violet is on a clear morning or at the brink of dusk several days after a rain shower. Violet leaf oil, which is available as a concrete and an absolute, is obtained primarily from the leaves of the Victoria violet, which do not lend themselves to mass production. Perhaps this is why I cherish this oil, because it takes time and great care to capture its essence. Luckily, you need just a touch to lend its scent to a synergy, and this makes up for its high price.

The aroma of violet leaf affords a nearly instant sense of serenity and comfort deep in the core of your heart. The flower, presented to Jupiter by the virginal Greek nymphs of Iona, has stood as the symbol of modesty and simplicity. But how nature fools us once again, giving us such a seductive odor in this unpretentious plant. "Shrinking," indeed! Through the scent of violet alone one may speak openly, "Gently come hither."

Violet leaf may cause skin irritation in dermatologically sensitive individuals. A maximum of 1 to 2 drops is recommended in 1 to 2 teaspoons of a base product or in a bath.

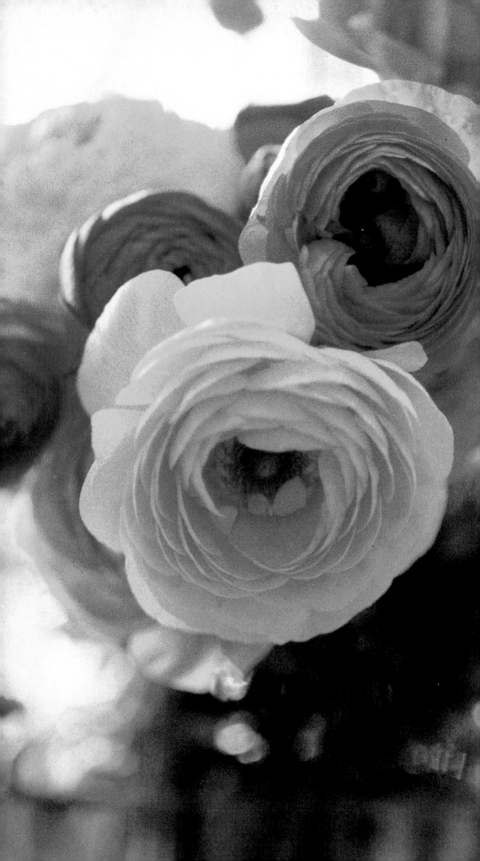

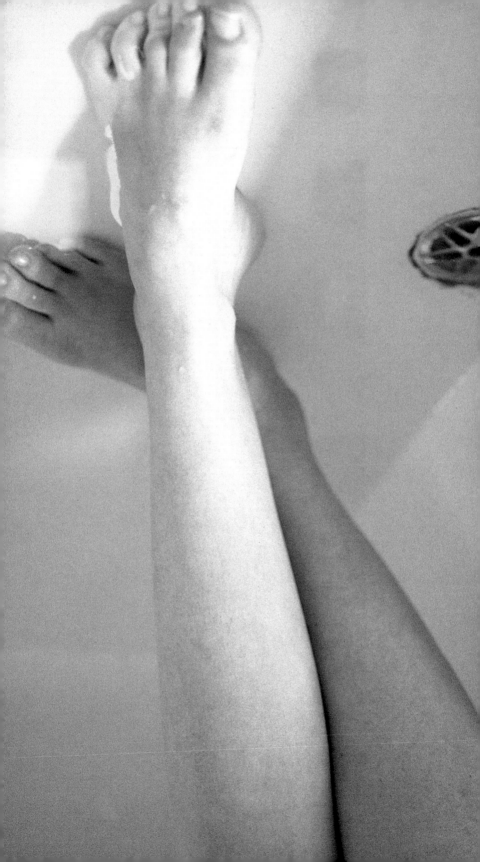

resources

The following companies and individuals are committed to supplying superior aromatic products, as well as professional training and consultation.

PUBLISHERS

Aromatherapy Today
International Aromatherapy Journal
email: jkerr@aromatherapytoday.com
website: www.aromatherapytoday.com
See also Springfields Aromatherapy.

Essential Oil Resource Consultants
2 ruelle du Teatre Butet
53240 St. Germain le Guillaume,
France
Tel/Fax: (33) 2 43 02 77 28
email: essentialorc@compuserve.com
You can purchase here the
Aromatherapy Database compiled by
Bob Harris. You can purchase the
International Journal of Aromatherapy
at website:
harcourt-international.com/journals/ijar

Aromatherapy Registration Council
Professional Testing Corporation
1350 Broadway 17th Floor
New York, NY 10018
Tel: (212) 356-0660
website: www.ptcny.com
Organization set up to make available
a National Examination and Registry
for Aromatherapists and
Aromatologists in the U.S.

Aroma History Archives
Sharon Gibson, RN, NCTMB
69 Harrison Drive
Willingboro, NJ 08046
Tel: (609) 835-4918
Fax: (609) 835-0181
email: aroma2@earthlink.net
Dealer in rare books and provider
of aromatherapy and essential oil
history classes.

Allured Publishing:
One of the Largest Publishers of
Aromatic Research Periodicals
Resource Directory
362 Schmale Road
Carol Stream, IL 60188-2787
Tel: (630) 653-2155
Fax: (630) 665-2699
email: customerservice@allured.com
Sudha Bhatt, Managing Editor,
Journal for Essential Oils Research
email: sbhatt@allured.com
Jeb Allured-Gleason, Managing Editor,
Perfume & Flavorist
email: jallured@allured.com
Melinda Taschetta-Millane,
Managing Editor, *Skin Inc.*
email: taschetta-millane@allured.com
website: www.SkinInc.com

American Botanical Council
PO Box 201660
Austin, TX 78720-1660
Orders: (800) 373-7105
Tel: (512) 331-8868
Fax: (512) 331-1924
email: custserv@herbalgram.org
Publisher of *Herbalgram* and *Herbal
Educational Catalog*, a mail-order
catalog of hard-to-find books.

IMPORTERS, EXPORTERS,
MANUFACTURERS, AND
PRODUCERS

Essential Aura Aromatics
Kent McKay, CEO
3688 Glen Oaks Drive
Nanaimo, British Columbia
V9T 5A1 Canada

Tel: (250) 758-9464
Fax: (208) 361-8940
email: info@essentialaura.com
website: www.essentialaura.com
Specialized distiller of organic and
ethically wildcrafted therapeutic
essential oils, with a focus on ecologically sustainable production practices
and the development of community
grower cooperatives in the Pacific
Northwest and Latin America.
Note: Aromatherapeutic grade oils
introduced in this book can be pur-
chased through this source at
www.essentialaura.com or phone
(250) 758-9464. Oils may be pur-
chased separately or in individual
"kits" based on the Basic oils and the
Sensuous oils.

A Woman of Uncommon Scents, Inc.
Importer of Extraordinary Essential
Oils
PO Box 103
Roxbury, PA 17251
Tel: (800) 377-3685
Fax: (717) 263-6347
email: rshapiro@epix.net
website:
www.awomanofuncommonscents.com
An importer of therapeutic quality
organic and wildcrafted essential oils
bought direct worldwide from farmers
and distillers. Sales are wholesale
only.

**American Herbalists Guild—A
Professional Association of Herbal
Practitioners**
1931 Gaddis Road
Canton, GA 30115
Tel: (770) 751-6021
Fax (770) 751-7472
email: ahgoffice@earthlink.net
website: www.americanherbalist.com

Aroma Trading Limited
John Black, CEO
Unit 14 Chapel Farm
Hartwell, Northampton NN7 2EU
United Kingdom
Phone: (44) 1808 511881
Fax: (44) 1908 566988
email: johnblack@aromatrading.com
website: www.aromatrading.com
Producer and exporter of pure, gen-
uine, and organic essential oils and
floral hydrolats.

The Essential Oil Company
Robert Seidel, CEO
1719 SE Umatilla Street
Portland, OR 97202
Orders: (800) 729-5912
Tel: (503) 872-8735
Fax: (503) 872-8767
email: office@essentialoil.com
website: www.essentialoil.com
Producer of essential oils, distributor
of Wilde and Company Forasoles™,
manufacturer of the Portable Home
Distiller, and developer of the Native
Essential Oil Network (NEON).

Florial
Alain Durante, CEO
42 Chemin des Aubepines
06130 Grasse, France
Tel: (33) 493 778819
Fax: (33) 493 778878
email: info@florial.com
website: www.florial.com
Producer and exporter of therapeutic
organic products that bear the
Agriculture Biologique (AB) symbol
and are controlled by ECOCERT.

Kim Manley
2999 Dillon Beach Road
Dillon Beach, CA 94929
Tel: (707) 878-2980
email: mail@kmherbals.com
website: www.kmherbals.com
Private-label manufacturer of organic
aromatherapy and botanical personal
care products.

Springfields Aromatherapy
Quality essential oils
email: jkerr@springfieldsaroma.com
website: www.springfieldsaroma.com

Essentially Oils
Charles Wells, CEO
Contact Tim Vaughan
8-10 Mount Farm, Churchill
Chipping Norton, Oxfordshire OX7 6NP
United Kingdom
Tel: (44) 1608 659544
Fax: (44) 1608 659566
email: sales@essentiallyoils.com
website: www.essentiallyoils.com
Distributors of quality essential oils and
aromatherapy products and publishers
of a monthly newsletter.

Boston Jojoba Company
PO Box 771
Middleton, MA 01949
Toll Free: (800) 256 5622
Tel: (978) 777-9332
Fax: (978) 777-1001
email: bob@bostonjojoba.com
website: www.bostonjojoba.com
Jojoba growers and providers of
HobaCare™, 100% Pure Golden Liquid
Jojoba.

Quintessence Aromatics, Inc.
PO Box 536
107 Main Street
Marsing, ID 83639
order: (800) 527-6467
Tel: (208) 896-417/ (208) 896-5073
Fax: (208) 896-4348
email: qai@w-idaho.net
website:
www.quintessencearomatics.com
www.jasmins.com
E.O.b.b.d.-certified therapeutic essential oils, and quality base oils.

Leyden House Limited
Gerry and Ann MacCarthy, CEOs
200 Brattleboro Road
Leyden, MA 01337
Orders: (800) 754-0668
Tel: (413) 772-0858
Fax: (413) 772-8858
email: leydeneo@javanet.com
website: www.leydenhouse.com
Designer and distributor of the Essential
Air™ professional cool air diffuser.

Quintessence Aromatics Canada
PO Box 20057
Saskatoon, SK S7L 7K9
Canada
Tel: (306) 382-3200
Fax: (306) 382-3245
email: quintessencearomatics
@sk.sympatico.ca
website: www.aromatherapie.net
E.O.b.b.d.-certified therapeutic
essential oils and training.

The Institute of Aromatic Medicine
Shirley Price, CEO
Robert Stephen, Registrar
Aromed House
66 Upper Bond Street
Hinckley, Leicestershire LE10 1RS
United Kingdom
Tel: (44) 1455 615503
Fax: (44) 1455 615054
email: ShirleyPriceAroma@
compuserve.com

**Canadian Federation
of Aromatherapists**
Jan Benham, President
843479 Oxford Road, 84 RR3
Lakeside, Ontario NOM 2G0
Canada
Toll-free Tel: (888) 340-4445
Tel: (519) 475-9038
Fax: (519) 475-9078
email: cfa@sympatico.ca

National Association for Holistic Aromatherapy
2000 2nd Avenue, Suite 206
Seattle, WA 98121
Orders: (888) ASK-NAHA
Tel: (206) 256-0741
Fax: (206) 770-5915
email: info@naha.org
website: www.naha.org

International Federation of Aromatherapists (IFA)
Stamford House
2-4 Chiswick High Road
London W4 1TH
United Kingdom
Tel: (44) 1817 422605

The Register of Qualified Aromatherapists
PO Box 3431
Danbury, Chelmsford
Essex CM3 4UA
United Kingdom
Tel: (44) 1245 227957
Fax: (44) 1245 222152

ORGANIZATIONS AND INDIVIDUALS

The Australasian College
Dorene Petersen, Principal and CEO
530 First Street, Suite A1
PO Box 57
Lake Oswego, OR 98034
Orders: (800) 487-8839
Tel: (503) 635-6652
Fax: (503) 636-0706
email: achs@herbed.com
website: www.herbed.com
A state-licensed career school offering a range of programs in aromatherapy, herbal medicine, homeopathy, and related subjects by distance education and residential classes.

The International Institute of Traditional Herbal Medicine & Aromatherapy
Principal: Gabriel Mojay MRQA, MBACC, MRSS
35 California Road, Mistley, Essex CO11 1JA, England
Tel: (44) 1206 393465
email: info@aromatherapy-studies.com
website: www.aromatherapy-studies.com
The Institute offers a variety of accredited training courses at both Diploma and advanced levels. Representative of Materia Aromatica Certified organic essential oils.
Tel: (44) 207 207 3461
email: info@organic-essentialoils.com
website: www.materia-aromatica.com

Purple Haze Lavender Ltd.
180 Bell Bottom Road
Sequim, WA 98382
Tel: (888) 852-6560
website: www.purplehazelavender.com
Certified organic lavender and lavender products.

The Atlantic Institute of Aromatherapy
Sylla Sheppard-Hanger, L.M.T., Founder-Director
16018 Saddlestring Drive
Tampa, FL 33618
Tel: (813) 265-2222
email: Sylla@AtlanticInstitute.com
website: AtlanticInstitute.com
Offers self-directed courses and publishes *The Aromatherapy Practitioner Reference Manual* and other related resources.

The Aromatic Plant Project
PO Box 225336
San Francisco, CA 94122-5336
Tel: (415) 464-6785
email: info@aromaticplantproject.com
website: www.aromaticplantproject.com
Non-profit organization founded by
Jeanne Rose. Mission is to encourage
the distillation and growing of true
essential oil plants and the production
of hydrosols in the U.S.

Analytical Intelligence
10 Mount Farm
Junction Road, Churchill
Chipping Norton, Oxfordshire
OX7 6NP United Kingdom
Tel: (44) 1608 659522
Fax: (44) 1608 659566
Conducts independent, advanced
analysis of oils by GC/MS.

Shirley Price Aromatherapy Ltd
Essentia House, Upper Bond Street
Hinckley, Leicestershire
LE10 1RS United Kingdom
Tel: (44) 1455 615466
Fax: (44) 1455 615054
email:
Shirleypricearoma@compuserve.com
Provider of accredited courses, supplier
of essential oils, and publisher of the
quarterly journal *The Aromatherapist.*

Dr. Bruce Berkowsky
email: DrBruceB@cnw.com.
website:
www.naturalhealthscience.com
Founder of Spiritual PhytoEssencing.
His books include: *Essential Oils
And The Cancer Miasm; Essential
Oils And Emotional Pain, Grief And
Dying; Berkowsky's Synthesis Materia
Medica of Essential Oils; 21st Century
Self-Care.*

Victoria Edwards
Aromatherapy Institute
and Research Center
PO Box 2354
Fair Oaks, CA 95628
Tel: (916) 965-7546
Fax: (916) 962-3292
email: victoria@leydet.com
website: www.leydet.com
Aromatherapist, consultant, educator,
and owner of Leydet Aromatics mail-
order business.

Kendra Grace
PO Box 662
Graton, CA 95444
Tel: (707) 829-0799
Fax: (707) 829-7806
email: kendra@naturesgeometry.com
website: www.naturesgeometry.com
Aromatherapist, formulator of
psycho-aromatherapeutic perfumes,
and designer and distributor of
Aromajewels™.

Nelly S. Grosjean N.D.
La Cheviche
13690 Graveson en Provence
France
Tel: 33 (0) 490-958158
Fax: 33 (0) 490-905078
email:
aromatherapy@nellygrosjean.com
website: nellygrosjean.com
Practitioner, international lecturer,
and founder of Laboratoire Vie'Arome.

Ixchel Susan Leigh
Therapeutic Alchemist, Vibrational
AromaTherapist
PO Box 498
Hampstead, NH 03841
Tel: (800) 688-8343.
email: ixchel@vibrational.com
website: www.vibrational.com
Book, *Aromatic Alchemy*. Vibrational
AromaTherapy courses, certification.

Krishna Madappa
The Essence of Life
7106 NDCBU
Taos, NM 87571
Tel: (505) 758-7941
email: essence@newmex.com
website: www.sacredoilsofkrishna.com
Educator, international speaker, and
producer and importer of essential oils
from the sacred plants of India and
New Mexico.

Dr. Robert S. Pappas
Essential Oil University, Inc.
2676 Charlestown Road, Suite #3
New Albany, IN 47150 .
Tel: (812) 945-5000
Fax: (603) 506-2563
website: www.essentialoils.org

Sandrine van Slee
Nectar Aromatherapy
130 West 11th Street, 3F
New York, NY 10011
Tel: (212) 243-3533
email: SandrineVS@aol.com
Certified aromatherapist, natural
perfumer, distributor for Janina
Sorensen.

Wild Herbs of Crete
Janina M. Sørensen, MSc, Medical
Herbalist, RN
Babis Psaroudakis, Botanist,
Masterdistiller
Tel/Fax: (45) 56480093
email: janinaherb@bigfoot.com
website: www.nature-helps.com/crete
Distillation of Cretan wildcrafted
herbs. Research, courses, education.

Peter Holmes, LAC, MH, AHG
Snow Lotus Aromatherapy
875 Alpine Avenue, Suite 5
Boulder, CO 80304
Tel: (303) 443-9289
Fax: (303) 443-6361
email: snowlotus@estreet.com
website: www.snowlotus.org

Mark Webb, B.Sc.D. Aroma DRM
PO Box 285
Blaxland NSW 2774
Australia
Tel/Fax: (612) 4727 6707
email: mark@bush-sense.com
website: www.bush-sense.com
Clinical aromatherapist, author of
Bush Sense, Australian essential oils
and aromatic compounds. Researcher
and supplier of Australian aromatics
(oils, hydrosols, herbals).

further reading

Advanced Aromatherapy
by Kurt Schnaubelt, Ph.D.
(Healing Arts, 1995)

The Ancient and Healing Art
of Aromatherapy
by Claire Hill
(Ulysses, 1997)

Aroma-Spa Therapy
by Anne Roebuck
(Anessence, 1995)

Aromatherapy A–Z
by Patricia Davis
(C.W. Daniel, 1999)

The Aromatherapy Companion
by Victoria Edwards
(Storey Books, 1999)

Aromatherapy for Healing the Spirit
by Gabriel Mojay
(Henry Holt, 1999)

Aromatherapy for Health Professionals
by Shirley and Len Price
(Churchill Livingstone, 1995)

Aromatherapy for Horses
by Caroline Ingraham
(Kenilworth Press, 1997)

Aromatherapy for the Healthy Child
by Valerie Ann Worwood,
(New World Library, 2000)

Aromatherapy in Midwifery Practice
by Denise Tiran
(Harcourt Brace, 1996)

Aromatherapy Massage
by Clare Maxwell-Hudson
(Dorling Kindersley, 1994)

Aromatherapy Pocketbook
by Kendra Grace
(Llewellyn Publications, 1999)

The Aromatherapy Practitioner
Reference Manual
by Sylla Sheppard-Hangar,
2 volumes (1994)

Aromatherapy Workbook
revised edition, by Marcel LaVabre
(Healing Arts, 1990)

The Art of the Bath
by Sara Slavin and Karl Petzke
(Chronicle Books, 1997)

The Art of Sensual Aromatherapy
by Nitya Lacroix with Sakina Bowhay
(Henry Holt, 1995)

Aveda Rituals
A Daily Guide to Natural
Health and Beauty
by Horst Rechelbacher
(Henry Holt, 1999)

Ayurveda and Aromatherapy
by Light Miller, N.D., and Bryan
Miller, D.C. (Lotus, 1995)

Bath Scents and **Health Scents**
by Alan Hayes
(Angus and Robertson, 1995)

The Book of Perfume
by Elisabeth Barillé and
Catherine Laroze
(Flammarion, 1995)

Botanical Drugs and Preparations
by R. C. Wren, F.L.S.
(C.W. Daniel, 1988)

Brother Cadfael's Herb Garden
Illustrated companion to Medieval
Plants and Their Uses
by Rob Talbot and Robin Whiteman
(Bulfinch Press, 1997)

The Chemistry of Essential Oils
by David Williams
(Micelle Press, 1997)

**The Chemistry of Essential Oils
and Artificial Perfumes**
by Ernest J. Parry
(Scott, Greenwood and Sons, 1921)

Clinical Aromatherapy in Nursing
by Jane Buckle (Singular, 1997)

Complete Aromatherapy Handbook
by Susanne Fischer-Rizzi
(Sterling, 1990)

The Complete Guide to Aromatherapy
by Salvatore Battaglia
(The Perfect Potion, 1996)

A Dictionary of Natural Products
4th edition, by George Macdonald
Hocking (Plexus, 1997)

Do It Yourself Pure Plant Skin Care
by Carol Stubbin,
(International Centre of Holistic
aromatherapy, 1999) Purchase at
email: perfect@thehub.com.au

Encyclopedia of Healing Plants
A Complete Guide to Aromatherapy,
Flower Essences and Herbal Remedies
by Chrissie Wildwood
(Jode Piatkus LTD, 1999)

Encyclopedia of Medicinal Plants
by Andrew Chevallier
(Dorling Kindersley, 1996)

**Essential Oil Safety: A Guide for Health
Care Professionals**
by Robert Tisserand and Tony Balacs
(Churchill Livingstone, 1995)

The Essential Oils
by Ernest Guenther, 6 volumes
(D. Van Nostrand, 1948–1952)

**Flower Oils and Floral Compounds
in Perfumery**
by Danute Pajaujis Anonis
(Allured, 1993)

Flower Power
by Anne McIntyre (Henry Holt, 1996)

The Fragrant Veil
Scents for the Sensuous Women
by Elisabeth Millar
(Llewellyn Publications, 2000)

From Flower to Fruit
by Anne Ophelia Dowden
(Ticknor and Fields, 1994)

The Garden of Life
by Navenn Patnaik
(Harper Collins, 1993)

Handbook of Perfumes and Flavors
by Dr. Olindo Secondini
(Chemical Publishing, 1990)

Hydrosols: The Next Aromatherapy
by Suzanne Catty
(Healing Arts Press, 2000)

The Healing Bath and **The Scented Bath**
by Maribeth Riggs
(Viking, 1996 and 1997)

The Healing Energies of Water
by Charlie Ryrie
(Journey Editions, 1999)

The Healing Garden
by Helen Farmer-Knowles
(Sterling, 1998)

Home Herbal
by Penelope Ody
(Dorling Kindersley, 1995)

Home Spa
by Manine Rosa Golden
(Abbeville, 1997)

Jitterbug Perfume
by Tom Robbins
(Bantam Books, 1984)

The Indian Materia Medica
by Dr. K.M. Nadkarni
(Popular Prakashan Pravate, 1976)

Indian Medicinal Plants
Mgr. B.D. Basu, 4 volumes
(Bishen Singh Mahendra Palsingh,
1993)

Love Scents
How your Natural Pheromones
Influence Your Relationships, Your
Moods, and Who You Love
by Michelle Kodis, Dr. David Moran,
and Deborah Houy
(Dutton Books, 1998)

Love Scents A Modern Herbal
by M. Grieve, volumes 1 and 2
(Dover, 1971)

A Natural History of the Senses
by Dianne Ackerman
(Vintage, 1990)

Perfume
by Patrick Suskind
(Washington Square Press, 1985)

Perfume Album
by Jill Jesse
(Robert and Krieger, 1974)

**Perfume and Flavor Materials
of Natural Origin**
by Steffen Arctander
(Allured, 1994)

The Perfume of Memory
by Michelle Nikly
(Arther A. Levine Books, 1999)

Perfumes, Splashes, and Colognes
by Nancy M. Booth
(Storey Books, 1997)

**Potter's New Cyclopaedia of
Botanical Drugs and Preparations**
by R.C. Wren, F.L.S
(C.W. Daniel, 1988)

**Reveal Your Glow, Brush Your Body
Beautiful**
by Donna Rae
(Earth Time Publications, 1999)

Scent and Psyche
by Peter and Kate Damian
(Healing Arts, 1995)

The Sensuous Garden
by Mantagu Don
(Simon and Schuster, 1997)

Scents and Scentuality
Aromatherapy and Essential Oils for
Romance, Love and Sex
by Valerie Ann Worwood
(New World Library, 2000)

Stories the Feet Have Told
by Eunice Ingham (1938)

belief in the power of the doctor's magic staff. The doctor then told him that the "magic" lay in the aromatic spices and herbs that filled the staff's handle. As the wayfarer had gripped the handle and leaned upon it for support, the essences had made their way upward through his hand, permeated his skin, and anointed his body with their healing powers.

Inscribed on one of the rings I wear is this quote from Rumi: "A mountain keeps an echo deep inside itself; that's how I hold your voice." The words speak to me daily and remind me of my own voice when I think it is lost to me. More significantly, they represent the spoken and unspoken intention of all the voices of my family, friends, and peers, alive and departed, who have loved me, supported me, celebrated me, encouraged my abilities, mourned my defeats, allowed me my frailties, renewed my faith when it waned, forgiven me when I disappointed them, and believed in the path I have chosen for my life.

My hope is that when you close the cover of this book, I have been able to plant in you the seeds of curiosity that will lead you to further explore the art and potential of aromatherapy. I ask you to respect, honor, and rekindle your celebration for this amazing planet so filled with the abundance of life, beauty, and mystery, and to never forget the immeasurable possibility of the human spirit.

May you find a way each day to wonder at the moon, sing to the sun, listen to the stars, and dance with the wind.

Aromatically yours,

Éva-Marie Lind

author's note

More than 500 years ago, Afghan poet and philosopher Rumi committed to writing his wondrous poetry of love and soul searching. Little
did he know that one of his stories would be added in time to the lore
of aromatherapy. It is the story of the wayfarer who was stricken with
an incurable malaise. One day in his travels, the wayfarer met a doctor

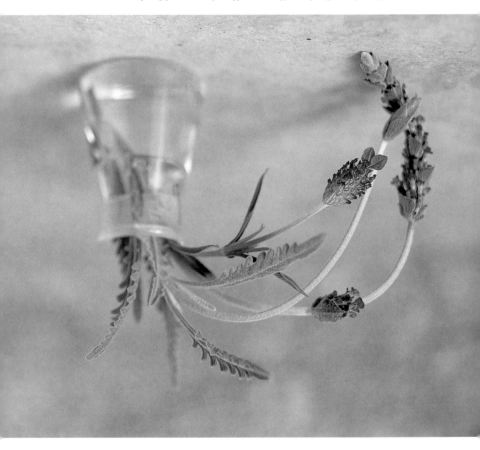

who gave him the gift of a walking staff with magical healing powers.
The doctor instructed the wayfarer to keep the staff close to his side as
he walked. Some weeks later, the wayfarer found himself completely
cured. Upon meeting the doctor again, he jubilantly announced his